FITNESS THROUGH

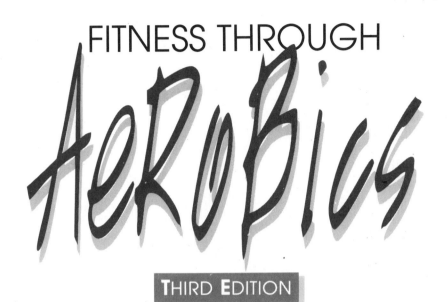

THIRD EDITION

Jan Galen Bishop

SOUTHERN CONNECTICUT STATE UNIVERSITY

GSP

Gorsuch Scarisbrick, Publishers

SCOTTSDALE, ARIZONA

Hexalite, Spenco, Sorbothane, Lycra, Supplex, Cardio Combat, Step Reebok, Walkman, Styrofoam, Dyna-bands, Therabands, Velcro, Betadine, and Reebok are registered trademarks.

Publisher	John W. Gorsuch
Editor	Nils Anderson
Consulting Editor	Robert P. Pangrazi
Developmental Editor	Gay L. Pauley
Production Manager	A. Colette Kelly
Production Editor	Carma Paden
Photography	William G. Nelson
Cover Design	Kevin Kall
Typesetting	ProType Graphics

Gorsuch Scarisbrick, Publishers
8233 Via Paseo del Norte, Suite F-400
Scottsdale, Arizona 85258

10 9 8 7 6 5 4 3 2 1

ISBN 0-89787-628-8

Copyright © 1989, 1992, and 1995 by Gorsuch Scarisbrick, Publishers

Printed in the United States of America.

Library of Congress Cataloging-in-Publication Data

Bishop, Jan Galen.
   Fitness through aerobics / Jan Galen Bishop — 3rd ed.
     p. cm.
   Previous eds. published with title: Fitness through aerobic dance.
   Includes bibliographical references and index.
   ISBN 0-89787-628-8
   1. Aerobic dancing.   2. Physical fitness.   3. Health.   I. Bishop, Jan Galen. Fitness through aerobic dance.   II. Title.
RA781.15.B58   1995
613.7—15–dc20   95-3078
                                                            CIP

Contents

Preface *vii*
Introduction *ix*

CHAPTER 1 — The Aerobics Look: Clothing and Equipment 1
Clothing 1
Equipment 6
Summary 7
Knowledge Tips 7

CHAPTER 2 — Fitness Components and Exercise Principles 9
Components of Fitness 9
Principles of Exercise 11
Summary 13
Knowledge Tips 13

CHAPTER 3 — The Aerobic Target Zone 15
Frequency 15
Time 16
Intensity 16
Summary 22
Knowledge Tips 23

CHAPTER 4 — Setting Goals and Reaching Your Dream 25
Step One: Establishing Your Fitness Goals 26
Step Two: Finding Motivation 27
Step Three: Choosing the Activity 28
Step Four: Measuring Your Progress 28
Step Five: Evaluating the Program and Your Goals 29

Summary   30
Knowledge Tips   30

CHAPTER 5

Warming Up and Cooling Down   31
Warm-Up   31
Cool-Down   43
Summary   44
Knowledge Tips   44

CHAPTER 6

Rhythmic Aerobics: Variations and Styles   45
The Aerobics Portion of Class   46
Techniques That Apply to All Rhythmic Aerobics   46
High-Impact Aerobics   47
Low-Impact Aerobics   48
Step Aerobics   49
Basic Steps for Step Aerobics   50
Aqua Aerobics   53
Circuit Aerobics   54
Slide Aerobics   55
Aerobics Videotapes   58
Summary   58
Knowledge Tips   58

CHAPTER 7

Body Toning Exercises   59
Frequency   60
Intensity   60
Time   60
Isometric and Isotonic Contractions   61
Technique for Body Toning Exercises   61
Summary   76
Knowledge Tips   76

CHAPTER 8

Body Toning Using Bands, Weights, and Water   77
Exercise Bands   78
Weights   83
Water   83

Summary   84

Knowledge Tips   84

CHAPTER 9

Exercises to Avoid   85

Summary   89

Knowledge Tips   89

Suggestions for Modifying or Correcting the Exercises to Avoid   89

CHAPTER 10

The Benefits of Aerobic Dance Exercise   91

The Metabolic Systems   92

The Cardiovascular System   93

The Respiratory System   95

The Skeletal System   95

The Muscular System   95

Other Systems   97

The Psychological Benefits of Exercise   97

Summary   98

Knowledge Tips   98

CHAPTER 11

Nutrition and Weight Control   99

Basic Nutritional Information   99

The Food Pyramid   102

Weight Control Information   103

Commonly Asked Questions   111

Summary   112

Knowledge Tips   112

CHAPTER 12

Care and Prevention of Injuries   113

Foot Injuries   114

Shin Injuries   115

Knee Injuries   115

Multiple Site Injuries   116

Heat-Related Injuries   117

Other Health Concerns   118

Commonly Asked Questions   119

Summary   121

Knowledge Tips   121

CHAPTER 13   Now That You're Fit . . .   123

Summary   125

Knowledge Tips   125

Bibliography   127

Glossary   131

Appendix   135

Muscles of the Body   136

Your Back and How to Care for It   137

Worksheets   139

1: Health and Fitness History   141

2: Summary Record Sheet   143

3: Calculating Your Target Heart Rate Range   145

4: Heart Rate Chart   149

5: Cardiorespiratory Fitness   151

6: Flexibility   159

7: Muscular Endurance   165

8: Healthy/Ideal Weight   169

9: Nutrition Awareness   171

Index   177

Preface

Aerobic dance exercise, once thought to be nothing more than a fad, now holds a prominent position in fitness programs throughout the United States. When Kenneth Cooper, M.D., kicked off the aerobics revolution in 1968 with his first book, *Aerobics,* he was not referring to aerobic dance. To him aerobics meant jogging, swimming, cycling, and other forms of aerobic exercise. In 1972, Jackie Sorensen took Cooper's passion for aerobic conditioning and combined it with music and dance. Since then, aerobic dance exercise has evolved into many styles, and today more than 24 million Americans find fitness through step, jazz, aqua, slide, and many other forms of aerobic exercise. Classes continue to overflow with new and veteran exercisers.

This enthusiasm for aerobic exercise has created a delightful dilemma. People who have never exercised before or who have had limited instruction in exercise are suddenly asking all kinds of questions about aerobics. The instructor faced with educating a gymnasium filled with people is in an environment that demands movement and motivating music, not talk. A well-informed and professional instructor certainly can educate as the class proceeds but is severely limited by time and acoustics.

This book was written to provide a solution to this dilemma. Students can read through vital information outside class; instructors can quickly clarify, reinforce, and supplement the information during class, leaving everyone enough time to enjoy a full aerobic workout.

The purpose of this book, then, is to place important exercise information, as it pertains to various forms of aerobic dance exercise, into the hands of participants. This knowledge will enhance the participants' ability to (1) understand the important relationship between regular exercise, health, and wellness, (2) perform exercises correctly, (3) maximize the training effect of exercise, and (4) take control of planning and executing a lifetime fitness plan.

The introduction and first four chapters contain the information needed to start an exercise program. They include suggestions on how to select clothing and equipment, how to use the basic principles of exercise, how to set goals, and how to monitor exercise intensity.

Chapters 5 through 8 delve into the specifics of exercise technique. Photographs and guidelines provide safe, effective techniques for the warm-up, aerobics, body toning, and cool-down portions of the class. The aerobics sections discuss low-, high-, and combination (high-low) impact and look at step, slide, and aqua (water) exercises. The chapters on body toning include strength and endurance exercises with and without equipment.

Chapters 9 through 12 examine *why* exercise is important, *how* to optimize the benefits of exercise, and *how* to exercise safely. Topics include the short- and long-range effects of exercise on the different systems of the body, injury prevention and care, nutritional guidelines for diet and exercise, answers to commonly asked questions, and discussions countering exercise myths. These chapters also include information on how to exercise with the added complication of pregnancy, asthma or diabetes, or back pain. The final chapter (13) takes a look at the programs available to anyone who makes a lifetime commitment to staying aerobically fit.

Each chapter opens with an overview and closes with a summary and a list of knowledge tips. Information critical to starting an exercise program is presented first; supplementary information follows. Key words, highlighted in bold throughout the book, are defined in a glossary at the back. Tear-out worksheets coinciding with information presented in the chapters are also located at the back of the book. These worksheets include a health and fitness questionnaire, training heart rate formulas, fitness tests, and nutrition awareness exercises, among others.

NEW TO THIS EDITION

Aerobic dance exercise has changed and grown at an exciting pace. New styles such as funk and combat aerobics are jumping into the market along with new innovations in step and slide aerobics. To keep pace with this changing aerobics arena, this third edition has been dramatically updated and improved. Here is a preview of some of the most significant changes:

1. Physical fitness in the 1990s is considered a part of overall wellness; the new introduction explains the relationship of aerobic dance exercise to wellness.

2. Updates on the shoe diagram and discussion reflect the fast-moving changes in technology.

3. The chapter on the aerobic target zone clarifies the rationale for two different heart rate formulas; the new worksheets contain examples of each.

4. A new chapter handles the wide variety of rhythmic aerobic exercises available today. Newcomers can learn basic step aerobics moves from easy diagrams. Explanations of low-, high-, and combination (high-low) impact aerobics have been expanded. Three new sections cover aqua, slide, and circuit aerobics.

5. Another new chapter updates the previous edition's information on bands and weights with new pictures and exercises and additional information on how to tone muscles in water.

6. Additional back exercises emphasize flexibility and strength.

7. Readers can now quiz themselves on how to fix the "exercises to avoid," self-checking with the answers at the end of the chapter.

8. A 12-inch bench step test has been added, since many classes now have step aerobics benches. The 16¼-inch step test has been retained for those who still wish to use bleachers.

9. Two versions of the curl-up test replace the sit-up test.

10. The book includes new discussions of back care and food labeling. Also, improvements in the nutrition worksheets make organizing the information easier. The summary worksheet now includes a place to list skin-fold measurements.

The information in this book is a synthesis of my experiences teaching at colleges, private clubs, instructor training/certification workshops, and conventions, plus knowledge and ideas I have gathered from instructors, professors, professional organizations, and, perhaps most importantly, students. These pages contain what I believe is the most pertinent information available. My hope is that this book will enable readers to more fully realize their exercise dreams.

ACKNOWLEDGMENTS

My sincere thanks to the following individuals, who read and offered suggestions regarding the third edition prospectus and manuscript: A. Lynn Berle, North Carolina State University; Dayna S. Brown, Morehead State University; Lisa Chaisson, Lamar University; Cissy Clark, Northeast Louisiana University; Mary L. Halverstadt, Lamar University; Anita Kissinger, Harrisburg Community College; Nancy McNamara, Broward Community College; Rob O'Connor, Broward Community College, South; Robert P. Pangrazi, Arizona State University; Kathleen Powell, Texas Tech University; Connie Reynolds, Utah Valley State College; Jacalyn Robert, Texas Tech University; Jodi M. Senk, University of Connecticut; Roland Schilder, Houston Community College; Peggy Smith, North Carolina State University; Carolyn Teague, Houston Community College; and Jean Teague, Houston Community College. The book is improved as a result of their constructive suggestions.

William G. Nelson and his assistant Christopher St. Johns are responsible for the fine photography and my sister Melissa Galen Bennie for the original artwork (shoe drawing). I'd also like to thank Melissa for her discriminating artistic eye during photograph selection. Pictured in those photographs are some very special people. I'd like to thank each of my models for helping bring the information in this book alive: Jessica Aman, Dara Elena Johnson, Teri So Dame, Patrick Decker, Ed Duclos, Rich Bishop, Carolanne M. Baker, and our newest little model, William "Beau" Baker V.

The GSP staff has been especially helpful and supportive in putting together a quality text. I'd like to thank Colette Kelly for her production expertise; the third edition is greatly improved thanks to her efforts. Gay Pauley has been my editor and friend (a tough combination) for over five years, and I have failed to thank her in either of the previous two editions. Thank you Gay! Your confidence and guidance have been invaluable. Finally, I must thank the most generous, understanding man in the world — thank you Rich.

INTRODUCTION

Aerobics, Wellness, and You!

You are the heart of the aerobics movement. Your well-being, your needs, your goals, your preferences … these are what should determine your workout. To be successful, you must take an active role in determining it. How? By combining what you know about yourself with the expertise of the instructor.

Too often we rely upon the expert to "fix" us, ignoring our role in the process. **Wellness**, a term first popularized in the 1980s, is about taking control of your personal well-being. Wellness includes mental, social, physical, intellectual, environmental, and spiritual health. By establishing a lifestyle that promotes wellness, you practice preventive medicine and enhance your quality of life.

Physical fitness is an important part of wellness, a part that promotes not only physical but also mental health. Joining an aerobic dance–exercise program is a giant step toward wellness. But blindly following the instructor is not enough. Strive to understand basic physical fitness concepts so that you can ask the right questions and can individualize your workout, now as well as later in life when your needs change. Experts are valuable teachers and guides, but only by combining your expertise with theirs will you find your optimal exercise program.

INDIVIDUAL DIFFERENCES

This book is about tailoring an aerobics program for you. Understanding the why and how of specific exercises enables you to make informed decisions about the exercises you want to include in your program. There is often more than one right way to achieve a goal. For instance, you can achieve the same cardiorespiratory health benefits from participating in dance exercise, step, or aqua (water) aerobics classes. Learning which exercises are interchangeable will help you design a well-balanced program.

The information in this book is based on sound research and on strategies and techniques practiced by numerous professionals. It is not, however, meant to be adhered to without consideration of your individual needs. Research tells us that the fastest a person's heart can beat is equal to 220 minus the person's age. Yet the maximum heart rates of some 20-year-old exercisers exceed 200 beats per minute, while others never reach 200. The formula is based on the average person and provides a good guideline—one from which adjustments should be made as needed.

A WELLNESS ATTITUDE

You can't control everything that happens to you, but you can control how you handle yourself in a situation. When you drive to school or work and can't find a parking space anywhere near the door, you have a choice: You can get irate or frustrated and complain to everyone you see for the next half hour, or you can welcome the opportunity to get some fresh air and start the day with an invigorating walk. Exercise is one of the few things over which you have almost complete control, and there are many wellness reasons for participating. You can

- Reduce your levels of stress, anxiety, and depression.

- Reduce your risk for physical ailments such as heart disease and stroke.

- Maintain a good ratio of fat and lean body mass by combining exercise and a balanced diet for a healthy and pleasant-looking physique.

- Lengthen your life span.

- Improve your quality of life at any age.

- Be uplifted and gain a renewed sense of energy.

AEROBIC EXERCISE

Any exercise promotes health; that's the good news. But certain kinds of exercise at certain levels of intensity provide you with the greatest health benefits. Aerobic exercise is key to enhancing cardiorespiratory fitness and lowering the risk of cardiovascular disease—the nation's number one killer. **Aerobic exercise** is any large-muscle, continuous, rhythmic activity. The word *aerobic* literally means "with oxygen" and only when oxygen is present in the muscle cells can fat be burned for energy. Many types of exercises are aerobic: brisk walking, jogging, cross-country skiing, rowing, cycling, swimming, and aerobic dancing are just a few.

Music has been used during exercise sessions for years, but in 1972 when Jackie Sorenson put together a routine of vigorous dance moves and music and called it aerobic dancing, she started one of the biggest fitness movements ever seen. Many dance exercise professionals believe the number of people involved in aerobic dance today is more than 24 million, although no one knows for sure. Since aerobic dance began, it has been shaped and changed by many innovative, creative instructors. Today aerobic dance includes high, moderate, low, and no impact styles influenced by jazz, hip hop, Latin American dance, modern dance, kick boxing, martial arts, and many other styles. In addition to regular aerobics classes, these styles can enliven step, double step, aquatic step, and aqua (water) aerobics classes. And, as well as other aerobics machinery—rowers, stair climbers, bikes, and the like—we now have the aerobics slide.

Besides being a good workout, aerobic dance exercise is also a social event. It is a great way to meet new people and a time you can set aside to spend with friends. Because the group setting is so important to motivation and having fun, instructors are challenged to create an aerobics workout that fits everyone's needs. One of the best ways to meet this challenge is to educate participants in modifying the moves to make them easier or more challenging, so that participants can work at their own level. A good instructor will flow from one level to another, demonstrating different levels and modifications of exercises. Some recent developments, such as step aerobics, make individualized exercising even easier: More skilled participants have higher steps and others have lower steps (or even no steps), thus individualizing the workout for each participant while everyone performs similar movements in unison with the instructor. This particular style of aerobics appeals to both men and women and has increased the number of coeducational classes.

SUMMARY

The explosion of variety in aerobic dance exercise keeps it fresh and exciting and enables people of all ages and at every fitness level to join in the fun. Innovative instructors and exercise-smart participants are riding the wave of wellness … and aerobic dance exercise is how they are doing it. Welcome back if you are experienced; welcome aboard if you a newcomer!

CHAPTER 1

The Aerobics Look: Clothing and Equipment

There are really two aerobics looks. One is toned, trim, and healthy. The other is stylish, fun, and faddish. The first can be achieved through regular exercise and proper nutrition. The second is much more immediate—

It can be bought!

Aerobic exercise classes have created a whole new fashion market. Today you can sweat in everything from classic grays to a wildly striped unitard.

People who exercise in clubs are usually the most fashion conscious. Most women wear a leotard (one or two piece) with tights or stretch shorts and matching socks, headbands, etc. Men wear either regular or stretch shorts with a T-shirt or stretch top.

Aerobic exercisers at colleges, YMCAs, recreation departments, churches, and schools often sport a more diverse dress. People there might wear sweat suits, shorts, T-shirts, or leotards and tights. Whichever look you choose, keep comfort and breathability foremost in your mind as you select each article of clothing. The remainder of this chapter provides specific information about articles of clothing and equipment associated with aerobic dance exercise.

CLOTHING

Shoes

Put your money where the stress is—invest in good shoes! Each time you jump, your feet absorb the impact of three times your body weight. The impact vibrations (shock) that cannot be absorbed by your arches are transmitted up your ankles, shins, knees, thighbones (femurs), hips, and spine and are eventually dissipated in the soft viscera (organs) in your trunk. The human body is wonderfully engineered to take stress, and with normal, routine activity, this system works beautifully. But when you add extra hours of jumping up and down to music, your body's shock-dissipating system needs some help. Shoes that provide good support and are well cushioned help absorb impact stress, make your workout more comfortable, and help prevent chronic stress injuries.

Athletic and dance shoes are designed to meet the specific needs of a physical activity. It is crucial to match the shoe to the activity. For example, soccer shoes have cleats so players can make quick changes of direction on grass. Running shoes have flared heels to provide lateral stability and prevent heel strike (bruising of the heel) when running straight ahead. Ballet and jazz shoes are soft and flexible so that dancers can land quietly, point their toes, and use all the foot positions required for dance. Using the wrong shoes can be calamitous. Just imagine running a race in ballet slippers, playing soccer in running shoes, or doing pirouettes in cleats!

Since aerobic dance exercise makes special demands on the body, the best shoes for this form of exercise are aerobic shoes (Figure 1.1). Scientists are continually studying the effects of aerobic dancelike movements on the feet. The information they have gathered has helped manufacturers design effective aerobic shoes.

You have to learn a whole new language to buy athletic shoes today. And like those of other fields, the technology and language of athletic shoes are constantly changing. On top of that each company will call a manufactured item by its own special brand name. In the following discussion I will sometimes mention brand-name features, but I am not promoting any one company. You must select a shoe that fits your foot and your needs.

Most aerobic shoes are designed to be lightweight, flexible, and shock absorbing. If you are a big person, bringing a lot of weight down on the shoe, a slightly heavier, sturdier shoe may be better than a light shoe.

On the bottom of the shoe is the outersole. Most aerobic shoes come with a similar amount of tread, but if you will be exercising on carpet you may wish to choose a shoe with a smoother tread, which will pivot more easily. Manufacturers are now cutting away the outersoles under the arch area in an attempt to save weight and materials. Since the arch area does not bear down on the ground with significant force, less outersole is needed here.

Most aerobic shoe companies are also grooving the outersole of the shoe to promote flexibility. Look on the bottom of the shoe for these grooves. A step shoe needs to have more flexibility than a high- or low-impact shoe.

The grooves on a step shoe may be deeper and wider in the forefoot, cutting partway into the midsole. The outersole should also have a flex point so that the shoe bends easily. Be sure that the bend of the shoe agrees with the bend in your foot when you are standing on the balls of your feet. Test the position of the bend by standing on the balls of your feet.

The midsole rests on top of the outersole and supplies most of the shock absorption. Many exercise steps involve landing on the ball of the foot first. To protect this part of the foot, an aerobics shoe must have extra forefoot padding. Manufacturers are using three shock-absorbing materials for midsole construction: EVA (ethyl vinyl acetate), compressed molded EVA, and polyurethane. The compressed molded EVA is an improved version of EVA and is therefore preferable to EVA. Polyurethane provides the best shock absorption but is slightly heavier and is therefore either not used or is used only sparingly. In addition to these effective synthetic foams, manufacturers have designed unique shock-absorption systems. For example, Avia uses a cantilever system, Nike an encapsulated air system, Asic an encapsulated gel, Rhyka encapsulated nitrogen, and Reebok a honeycombed inset called Hexalite. All of these methods add shock absorption and are particularly helpful in a high-impact shoe. Midsoles should also be flexible so that the foot can roll down comfortably with each step. Try bending the shoe with your hands.

Some low-impact shoes have extra shock absorption in the heel but not the forefoot. If you exercise in a mixed class or a step class, you will want the forefoot padding, so stay with a high-impact shoe or a good cross-trainer that provides support and cushioning in both areas.

Insoles are what your feet rest on inside the shoe, and along with the midsoles, they provide arch support and cushioning. The best insoles pull out so they can be aired between classes and replaced when worn out. (It is much less expensive to replace insoles than to buy a new pair of shoes.) You can upgrade your insoles by purchasing a pair made of compressed molded EVA, polyurethane, or neoprene. Spenco and Sorbothane both make excellent insoles. Some of the newest insoles include regular or graphite arch supports and materials that wick away moisture. If the shoe you purchased has a graphite arch (Reebok sells one), you probably don't want an insole of the same material. Orthotic wearers, check with your doctors concerning graphite arches built into the shoe—they may work against your orthotic. Insoles that come with aerobic shoes tend to break down quickly. If you decide to purchase a better insole, be sure to take your aerobic shoes and try the insole on in the shoe. Sometimes I have had to buy shoes one half-size

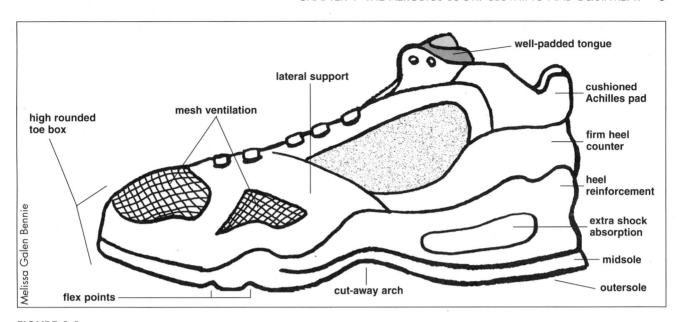

FIGURE 1.1
Aerobics shoe.

larger to accommodate these insoles. Regular washing of the insoles will allow them to breathe better and keep your feet cooler. You will be unclogging their pores so to speak.

Manufacturers have developed a variety of lacing systems. Some lacing systems allow for wider feet, some spread the tension, and some let you lock in the tension. Pump shoes let you custom fit the shoe by pumping air into the tongue or heel or surrounding areas after lacing. Some people enjoy this extra feeling of support; others find it an unnecessary expense. It is important, however, that both the tongue and the heel be well padded.

Lateral support stabilizes your foot during side-to-side movements and keeps your foot from twisting when you have your weight on the ball of your foot. Look for lateral support straps that run from the midsole up to the lacing. Beware of cosmetic stitching that looks like lateral reinforcement—try to find leather straps. Other sources of support are outsoles that wrap up the sides of the shoe and insoles and midsoles that curve up on the inside edges of the shoe to cradle the foot. Many shoes now also have a sock liner or sleeve that is attached to the tongue and sides of the shoe and wraps around your foot. A midcut shoe (as opposed to a low-cut or high-top shoe) provides added lateral support. Most cross-trainers and aerobic shoes come with a midcut. Walking and running shoes (activities that don't require side-to-side movement) come in low-cut styles.

To prevent side-to-side slippage in the heel, the shoe should have a firm, reinforced heel counter. The sole beneath the heel should extend out a little wider than the upper but should not have the flare of a running shoe.

The heel should also be well padded and notched so that your Achilles tendon is not irritated from frequent stepping and jumping.

Look at the leather (or other material) used for the upper (the body of the shoe). Firm leather and nylon materials provide support, while soft leathers stretch out and allow the feet to roll out over the soles. Some of the new uppers are made of sturdy synthetic washable leatherlike material (which lasts longer if hand washed). And finally, manufacturers are adding more mesh to their shoes to allow for air circulation (ventilation).

The main difference between high- and low-impact shoes is the amount of shock absorption you need. If you are doing a high-impact or mixed class, it is worth the extra money to get superior cushioning. Ideally a step shoe would be a little more flexible in the forefoot, since you are repeatedly stepping down onto a flexed foot. The bottom line is that any shoe that provides good lateral support, shock absorption, and flexibility in the midsole will work. If you are just getting started, you may want to opt for a good cross-trainer with these qualities. Walking (or running) shoes are not a good choice because they don't provide lateral support or extra forefoot padding.

When you buy a pair of shoes, which these days is a major investment, take them home and wear them indoors for an hour. If they don't fit properly they will still be clean and you can return them. If the shoe doesn't feel good without breaking it in, don't buy it. Try one brand after another until you find one that really fits.

When shopping for shoes, don't be afraid to ask the salesperson to tell you the difference between models. You may end up talking with the manager and learn a lot.

Sometimes you can save money by buying last year's shoe, especially if the only significant change in models is color.

Shoes that support the bones of the arch allow the ligaments that tie the bones together to relax. Shoes that don't support the arch stress the ligaments and tire the supporting muscles. Poor arch support can make your feet ache by the end of the day or even by the end of class. In addition to wearing supportive shoes, you need to build the strength of your arch muscles. Exercises done with your toes such as picking up marbles, gathering a towel toward you, and pushing the towel away are all effective ways of strengthening your arches.

Feet with significant mechanical or structural abnormalities such as very high arches, flat feet, or feet that tend to pronate (roll in) or supinate (roll out) often need more support than ordinary shoes can provide. In addition to making your feet ache, these abnormalities can cause impact vibrations to be sent up the legs on an angle. Vibrations repeatedly striking the knee at an angle can cause irritation on the inside or outside of the knee. Shinsplints, hip pain, and even lower back pain may originate from problems with the feet.

If you think your feet need extra support, consult a podiatrist, who might prescribe orthotics. Orthotics are custom-made plastic insoles that slip inside your shoe to provide form-fitting support. There are many kinds of orthotics. If you intend to use them for exercise, be sure to tell the podiatrist so that he or she will prescribe a sports orthotic; the more flexible sports orthotics give when you land from a jump. Orthotics are relatively expensive, but they are as indispensable to bad feet as eyeglasses are to bad eyes.

If you are just starting out in aerobic dance exercise and don't have aerobic or cross-training shoes, you are probably better off in a court shoe—those made for tennis, racquetball, etc.—than in a running shoe. Running is a very different activity from aerobic dance exercise: Running is unidirectional, aerobics multidirectional. Runners land near the heel of the shoe and need protection from heel strike; aerobic exercisers land primarily on the balls of their feet and need forefoot protection. The wide, flared heel that provides lateral stability for running allows too much side slippage during lateral aerobic dance movements. Furthermore, running shoes have a heavy tread designed for dirt and tar, not wood or carpeted surfaces. A court shoe has better heel construction for aerobic dance exercise, since it is designed for quick changes of direction. However, it is not cushioned enough, especially in the ball of the foot, for repetitive jumping. You may want to begin taking classes in a court shoe with an upgraded insole and then shop for an aerobic shoe.

When you are ready to buy aerobic shoes, use the following set of questions as a guide for selecting quality shoes:

1. Have I tried on at least three different brands, and does this brand feel the best on my feet? (Be sure you are wearing the same kind and number of socks you wear for class.)

2. Do these shoes have molded compressed EVA or the equivalent in the midsole for shock absorption?

3. Does the added shock-absorption system feel natural when I'm performing aerobic dance–exercise steps?

4. Is the heel counter firm? Does the heel fit snugly? Is the heel padded and notched at the top?

5. Does the insole come out for easy airing, washing, and replacement? Does the shoe still fit with my upgraded insoles or orthotics in place?

6. Can I bend the shoe easily (flexible midsole, outersole grooves, flex point, etc.)?

7. Is the toe box wide enough for my foot when I put weight on the ball of my foot and jump forward and backward?

8. Does the shoe provide lateral support (sock liner, wrapped outersole, support straps from the midsole to laces, etc.)?

9. Do I feel support through the arches?

10. Is the shoe well ventilated (toe box holes, mesh)?

11. Are these the correct shoes for the activities I do (high impact, mixed, low impact, step, cross training, proper tread, etc.)?

12. Are these shoes the best buy? Quality shoes often cost more but last longer and provide better support.

Once you've found the perfect pair of shoes, wear them, enjoy them, and keep an eye on wear and tear—even the best pair of shoes will wear out eventually. When your shoes are no longer supplying support and cushion, throw them out and start again. Of course by then you'll need a new technolanguage update!

Socks

Socks prevent blisters and calluses by reducing the friction between your shoes and the skin on your feet. For extra protection, wear two pairs of socks. The inner socks, which may be the feet on exercise tights, should be thinner than the outer socks. The socks slide across each other and further reduce the friction on your skin.

If you have sensitive feet or if you are planning a long day at a workshop or competition, you can further reduce friction by putting baby powder between your pairs of socks or by applying petroleum jelly to your feet. To prevent soreness when you are breaking in a new pair of shoes, place bandages or tape over sensitive areas such as the back of your heels and the outside of your little toes.

Socks also absorb perspiration, keeping your feet dry and helping prevent itching, cracking, and athlete's foot. Some of the newer acrylic or polyester blend socks effectively wick moisture away from your skin. All-cotton socks may also work for you. They are very good at absorbing moisture, but they also tend to hold that moisture next to your skin. When colored socks get wet (sweat soaked), the dye may irritate your skin. White socks are recommended next to the skin, but colored socks may be worn over white socks for style.

Tights

Tights come in a variety of weights and colors. Stay with light- to medium-weight tights and add sweat pants or warm-up socks if the room is cool. That way, you can peel off layers as you warm up.

Exercise tights supply support and shape to legs. They also provide nice coverage while you are performing exercises in a variety of positions in close quarters. Tights can be purchased with or without feet or with stirrups. Stirrup tights come down around the arch of the foot, but the toe and heel are cut out. Be sure that the stirrup is broad enough to stay flat under your foot and doesn't have heavy seams that will bother your arch. Some people find it more comfortable to put the stirrup under socks, others like it over socks. If you don't like stirrups or feet, you can purchase tights that are hemmed at the ankle, below the knee, or above the knee like shorts.

Women should be sure to purchase exercise tights or running pants because regular nylons trap heat and moisture and run too easily. There is considerable variation among brands, so check the sizing charts. Look for a cotton-aerated crotch, which helps prevent moisture build-up and infections. Both men's and women's exercise tights are now available at sporting goods stores and most department stores. To add pizzazz to your wardrobe you can buy shiny or patterned tights in a rainbow of colors. Look for materials that allow your skin

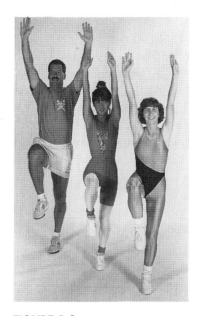

FIGURE 1.2
Aerobics clothing today offers a wide variety of styles, colors, and patterns.

to breathe. Lycra blends such as cotton-lycra and a newer material called Supplex (a nylon-lycra combination that wicks moisture away) are very popular.

Leotards

Leotards that used to come only in black and pink are now available in a myriad of colors, patterns, and styles. You can dress in neon colors, bright stripes, leopard spots . . . in French cuts, capped sleeves, two-piece sets, T-shirts and suspenders, or a unitard that goes on like a new layer of skin. Adding a brief over the top of a unitard adds color and is functional, too, as briefs keep the crotch from sagging and cover sweat lines. Leotards are a popular choice of attire for aerobic dance–exercise classes for several reasons. They allow for complete freedom of movement and are made of breathable materials so that heat is easily dissipated. Because they conform to the lines of the body, both participant and instructor can easily check body alignment.

Select leotards that are comfortable to move in. Try bending over in them as well as stretching upward and to the side. Make sure the straps will stay up and the T-shirt will stay down in a two-piece suspender style. A leotard that rides up can be irritating and a nuisance if you have to keep pulling it down. Leotards with high cuts are comfortable with tights but may be uncomfortable if worn under shorts without tights. Leotards that are too short in the body will pull up and can become painful around the legs. Check the fabric and allow for shrinkage, especially if you are going to machine wash and dry it.

Try on different styles. Just like regular clothing, different styles are made for different builds. For example, vertical stripes can be slimming, while different-colored bottoms, tops, and belts accentuate a waistline.

Quality fabrics wear for a long time. Other fabrics lose their color after a few washings. Check the stitching—poor stitching unravels in the wash.

Shorts

There are three kinds of shorts to consider. Very popular today are the stretch shorts that are form fitting and can be worn with a leotard or T-shirt. These provide excellent range of motion, breathability, and coverage. Another possibility is running shorts, which have attached undergarments so that the leg can be cut higher and wider to allow freedom of movement. Finally, regular leisure shorts are fine as long as they are cut wide enough in the legs and have an elastic waist. If you are wearing shorts without a leotard or tights, think about the different positions you'll be in during class (aerobics, body toning, and stretching) and make sure you are getting the coverage you want!

Undergarments for Women

The fabric in some leotards provides enough support for smaller-breasted women but not enough for most women during a jumping activity such as aerobic dancing. Sports bras provide extra support and are elastic so that you can breathe and move with ease. The seams, if there are any, are on the outside of the cup to prevent nipple abrasion, and the straps come in both regular and T-back styles. If a woman is pregnant or breast-feeding, a good bra is a must; maternity stores often carry bras suitable for exercise.

Warm-Up Socks

Traditionally, dancers wore warm-up socks to keep their legs warm while they rehearsed and warmed up in old, drafty theaters. Although conditions are not usually as inclement today, warm-up socks are still useful for getting the leg muscles warmed up for stretching and vigorous exercise. Some people find that the added warmth helps alleviate shinsplint pain. It is also wise to push warm-up socks down once you are warm so that your legs don't overheat. The short warm-up socks worn around the ankles were created for a fashion look and

serve no functional purpose. Warm-up socks can be purchased in several lengths and weights.

Belts

Dancers introduced the belt to their exercise attire as a functional tool. A belt can focus a person's attention on proper torso alignment. Instructors also may clip a battery pack for their headset microphone to a stretch belt. Today, most belts are purchased as a fashion accessory. Be sure the belts you choose allow for easy breathing and that they don't cut into you when you lie on your back for floor exercises.

Dangerous Clothing

Rubber and plastic suits prevent normal body cooling; dehydration and dangerous heat stress may result. The large weight losses observed after exercising in a rubber suit can be attributed to large fluid losses. As soon as the body is properly rehydrated, the weight will return. No positive health benefit is achieved with the use of these suits. Plastic wraps (cellophane) trap heat the same way rubber suits do and should be avoided for the same reasons.

Restrictive clothing that interferes with breathing must be avoided. Exercise demands oxygen and causes deeper, faster breathing. Restrictive clothing (such as belts, tight-fitting shorts, etc.) may result in shallow, inadequate breathing and can lead to fainting.

. . . .

EQUIPMENT

Mats

A good mat is easy to transport, clean, and store, and it has enough cushioning to keep you from feeling the floor during exercise. Some people are very happy working with a towel or a square of carpet; others prefer more cushioning. Some mats fold up to form a gym bag.

Weights

Weights can be effectively used by people who want to increase their muscular strength and endurance during aerobic dance exercise. Weights should be used only by individuals exercising at the intermediate or advanced level who have no history of joint problems such as arthritis, bursitis, ligament damage, or knee surgery.

They are available as hand-held weights, wrist weights, and ankle weights. If you have a tendency to clench hand-held weights, your arm may tire and cramp during the workout. Wrist weights allow you to relax your hands. When weight is at the end of your arm or leg, you must work harder to move it than if it is closer to your elbow or knee. Wrist and ankle weights that stretch can be pushed partway up your arm or leg to lighten the load when you first start and then may be moved down to your wrist or ankle when you are ready to handle the full weight. The weights come in a variety of sizes ranging from one-half to three pounds. See Chapter 8 for greater detail on the use of weights.

Exercise Bands

Regular, heavy-duty office rubber bands, specially produced exercise bands, cables with handles, or surgical tubing can be used as exercise bands. Their purpose, like weights, is to add resistance to strength exercises for individuals at the intermediate or advanced level. Anyone with previous joint injury or anyone who develops joint pain should not use the bands. Bands come in different widths and thicknesses. The wider or thicker the band, the more difficult it is to stretch. Some exercises require long bands that may be referred to as double bands. You can buy bands in different lengths. Exercise bands are used only during the body toning portion of aerobic dance exercise. See Chapter 8 for specific exercises.

Steps (Benches)

Steps or benches are platforms on which individuals step up and down. They are sold commercially, or you can build your own. Be sure the bench is stable and has a nonslip surface. You should start with a low bench (four inches) and work your way up to higher benches. You should never be stepping up on a bench that causes you to have less than a 90-degree bend under your knee. Stackable benches should fit snugly together and provide gradual increases in height. See Chapter 6 for details on step aerobics.

Pulse Readers

You can find your pulse easily by placing your fingers over your carotid or radial artery (Chapter 3), but if you like gadgets, you can purchase an electronic pulse reader. Unfortunately, the inexpensive ones that slip over your finger or clip onto your earlobe are generally unreliable and inaccurate. For about $150 to $200 you can purchase a more accurate heart rate monitor. These monitors have electrodes mounted on a band that wraps around the chest. Since the electrodes must touch skin, these monitors are difficult to wear with one-piece leotards. This type of monitor is most often used with cardiac patients or for research purposes.

SUMMARY

Although aerobic dance exercise has introduced a style of dress all its own, to get started all you really need is a pair of shoes that provide good support and a set of clothes that allow you to move, breathe, and sweat freely.

KNOWLEDGE TIPS

1. Wear nonrestrictive, comfortable clothing that allows you to sweat freely. Wear supportive undergarments.

2. Wear socks, tights, or both to prevent blisters and to absorb moisture.

3. Try on exercise clothing before purchasing it. Allow for shrinkage. Make sure that straps will stay in place while exercising.

4. Select aerobics shoes that have good cushioning and support.

5. Use weights and exercise bands only if you are free from joint injury and have attained at least an intermediate level of fitness. Start with light weights and easy resistance bands.

CHAPTER 2

Fitness Components and Exercise Principles

COMPONENTS OF FITNESS

Exercising for health is different from training for competition. To fine-tune your performance for competition you have to train long hours at high intensities. You may also have to place your body in mechanically difficult positions. For example, volleyball players and weight lifters drop into deep knee positions, which place stress on their knee ligaments. Gymnasts constantly hyperextend their backs, placing pressure on their vertebral discs, and pitchers risk injuring their elbows when they throw curve balls. The motivation for such intense practice and performance comes from a deep-seated drive to excel and a desire to win recognition and awards.

Many positive outcomes are associated with competition—health can even be one of them. However, a higher risk of injury is associated with high-intensity training. It may also surprise you to learn that not all highly trained competitors are physically fit. For example, some excellent golfers and baseball players carry extra pounds of fat and lack good cardiorespiratory conditioning.

When you exercise for health, you train at a more moderate intensity, which optimizes the physiological and psychological benefits of exercise and at the same time limits the risk of injury. The idea of exercising until you drop or killing yourself to get fit is wrong. Lifetime fitness is built on activities that are enjoyable and, when done correctly, free from pain.

There are five health-related components of physical fitness: cardiorespiratory endurance, body composition, flexibility, muscular strength, and muscular endurance. Any improvement in these five areas will improve your health. (Sometimes muscular strength and endurance are considered one component, making the total number of health-related components four.) There are also six skill-related components of fitness: coordination, agility, balance, reaction time, power, and speed. (Sometimes kinesthetic awareness is included as a seventh component.) Since aerobic dance exercise is primarily concerned with developing and maintaining physical health, exercises that concentrate on the five health-related components are emphasized. This emphasis does not exclude the possibility of improving some of the skill-related components, especially coordination, agility, and balance.

Cardiorespiratory Endurance

Cardiorespiratory endurance is the ability to perform large-muscle movements over a sustained period of time. Defined another way, it is the ability of the circulatory (heart, blood, blood vessels) and respiratory systems to deliver fuel, especially oxygen, to the muscles during continuous exercise. Fit individuals have a heart-lung capacity that allows them to persist in physical activity for relatively long periods of time without undue fatigue. (The terms cardiovascular endurance and cardiorespiratory endurance are often used interchangeably. The latter will be used in this text because it reflects the important relationship between the respiratory and circulatory systems.) Cardiorespiratory endurance is improved during the aerobic portion of the exercise class. Some of the health benefits associated with cardiorespiratory endurance include a stronger heart, improved circulation to the heart, increased oxygen transportation by the blood, a lower risk of coronary heart disease, a better chance of surviving a heart attack, a decreased level of blood fat (cholesterol), an increased level of high-density lipoproteins (HDL), a lowered resting heart rate, lower blood pressure, and a better chance of living a longer, healthier life.

Body Composition

Body composition refers to the relative amounts of lean body mass and fat in your body. **Lean body mass** includes bones, muscles, and connective tissue. **Fat** includes subcutaneous fat (the fat deposits stored between the muscles and the skin) and intramuscular fat

(the fat stored within the muscles). The percentage of fat you have can be measured several ways, including the skin-fold technique and underwater weighing (Chapter 11). A certain amount of fat is essential for health. Too high or too low a percentage of fat is unhealthy.

Body composition can be changed by decreasing the amount of fat, increasing the amount of lean body mass, or both. You can change your body composition through a sound diet and exercise program. Fat (along with carbohydrate) is metabolized during aerobic exercise, while muscle (lean body mass) can be added through strength training exercises. Increasing muscle mass has the added benefit of increasing your resting metabolic rate, which means your body is burning more calories while at rest. This can help you maintain a healthy weight after a weight-loss diet.

Maintaining an ideal body composition reduces the risk of coronary heart disease, makes you look and feel better, and increases your body's work capacity.

Flexibility

Flexibility is the ability to move a joint through its full range of motion. Muscles, tendons, ligaments, and bone structures all limit a joint to a normal range of motion. Loss of function occurs when a joint is too loose or too tight. When muscles and tendons tighten and shorten, the range of motion in the joint is restricted. Simple tasks such as turning in a car seat to check traffic or picking something up off the floor can become difficult. When ligaments and tendons are overstretched or damaged, the joint becomes loose and dislocates easily. Strengthening the muscles around a joint may help stabilize a loose joint, or surgery may be required. (A physician should be consulted to provide advice on which exercises are appropriate for rehabilitating an injured joint.)

Working on flexibility by stretching during the warm-up and cool-down periods of an aerobics class helps maintain and improve range of motion. Health benefits associated with good flexibility include freedom of movement (which represents independence for older individuals), greater work efficiency, less risk of muscle or joint injury, and decreased chance of developing lower back pain.

Muscular Endurance

Muscular endurance is the ability of a muscle, or group of muscles, to apply a submaximal force repeatedly or to sustain a muscular contraction for a period of time. Leg lifts are an example of repeatedly applied force. Holding the leg in a raised position for 10 seconds is an example of a sustained contraction. During leg lifts, the muscles go through a range of motion while applying force. This is called an **isotonic contraction** and is an example of a dynamic contraction. During a dynamic contraction, muscle fibers lengthen and shorten. When the leg is held in one position the muscles are in an **isometric contraction.** During a sustained isometric contraction, muscle fibers neither lengthen nor shorten. Most body toning exercises are done using isotonic contractions, since these contractions strengthen the muscle through its entire range of motion. Isometric contractions strengthen a muscle in a particular position, which can be particularly useful for improving posture. People with high blood pressure should avoid isometric contractions, which can cause a rapid rise in peripheral resistance (blood pressure). The benefits of improving muscular endurance include less fatigue during regular activity, an increased ability to do work, and a reduced risk of injury.

Muscular Strength

Muscular strength is the ability of a muscle, or group of muscles, to exert force against a resistance. The number of pounds you can lift one time with your arms is a measure of maximal muscular strength. You can improve your muscular strength by lifting relatively heavy weights a small number of repetitions. Aerobic dance–exercise classes have traditionally placed more emphasis on endurance than on strength, but the addition of bands, small weights, weighted balls, and step aerobics has enabled participants to improve strength. A well-designed weight training program is the best way to further increase strength. Strength training, like endurance training, usually emphasizes isotonic contractions. The health benefits related to muscular strength include an increased ability to do work (particularly physically challenging work), a decreased risk of injury, and a decreased risk of back pain.

PRINCIPLES OF EXERCISE

As you work to improve or maintain your fitness level in each of the five health-related components of fitness, use the following principles of exercise to guide you.

The Principle of Overload

When the human body is stressed repeatedly over a period of time, it responds by adapting to the stress. Regular exercise stresses the body, which adapts by becoming stronger and more efficient. Another word for stress is overload. When the muscles, including the heart muscle, are overloaded or stressed more than normal amounts, fitness gains occur. This is the **principle of overload.** To improve flexibility, the muscle is overloaded by being stretched longer than its normal length. To improve strength, overload is achieved by increasing the amount of resistance against which the muscle normally moves. To increase muscular endurance, overload is accomplished by repeatedly performing a movement more times than normal or by holding an isometric contraction for a longer time than normal. To improve cardiorespiratory endurance, overload consists of placing a greater than normal demand on the heart and lungs through sustained aerobic activity.

When you overload you are temporarily increasing the intensity of an exercise. As your body adapts, you experience a training effect and the exercise becomes easier. To continue to improve your physical fitness, you have to continue to overload. For example, if you can normally do 10 push-ups, create an overload to the arm and chest muscles by doing 11 or 12. When 12 becomes easy, overload again by doing 13 or 14, and so on. When you reach your desired level of fitness you can stop overloading. To maintain your fitness level, continue to perform your new "normal" amount. Doing less than normal will result in deconditioning.

A minimum amount and intensity of exercise must be performed before fitness improvement begins. This minimum level of exercise is called the **threshold of training.** To improve your physical fitness, you must exercise above your threshold of training. The threshold of training for a beginner is relatively low. As you become more fit, your threshold of training will increase. However, beyond a certain amount of exercise, the benefits diminish and the risk of injury increases.

The optimal range of exercise is called the **fitness target zone.** The lower limit of the zone is the threshold of training; the upper limit is the maximum amount of exercise that is beneficial. The best-known target zone is the one for cardiorespiratory endurance. However, target zones exist for each of the health-related components of fitness.

Three variables are involved with locating and exercising in your target zones: the frequency with which you train (number of times per week), the intensity at which you train, and the amount of time you train per session. These three variables are often remembered by the acronym **"FIT"**—the "F" stands for **frequency,** the "I" for **intensity,** and the "T" for **time** (or **duration**). Each fitness component has optimal ranges for these three variables. For example, to condition at the threshold of training for aerobic endurance, you must exercise three times a week, at 50 percent of your heart rate reserve, for a minimum of 20 minutes. You can achieve overload by increasing the frequency to four times a week, by increasing the intensity to 60 percent of heart rate reserve, or by increasing the duration to 30 minutes.

The target zone for aerobic endurance is described in more detail in Chapter 3. The target zones for flexibility and muscular strength and endurance are described in Chapters 5 and 7. Each of these chapters will discuss how to adjust the frequency, intensity, and duration of your exercise so that you get the most out of aerobic dance exercise.

The Principle of Progression

The **principle of progression** is an extension of the principle of overload. Basically, this principle means that you should not increase overload too slowly or too rapidly. Too slow an increase will delay or prevent improvement. Too rapid an overload can make you really stiff and sore or may even result in injury. For the best results, beginners should start out near the threshold of training and gradually add frequency and time, and then intensity, while staying within the target zone. Many people fail to progress because they exercise too infrequently or because they don't exercise vigorously enough to reach their threshold of training.

The Principle of Individuality

Everyone is unique, and this includes people's responses to exercise. The **principle of individuality** holds that no two people react exactly the same way to exercise. Two men with the ability to lift the same amount of weight can have significantly different muscle circumferences. Two women eating the same diet, attending the same exercise class, and working out at the same intensity will lose inches or pounds in different places at different rates. This means that the only person you can really compare yourself to is yourself. Your rate of progress and the way you progress is unique to you.

Many fitness tests provide norms, averages, or percentiles for you to compare your scores against. These are helpful guidelines, but they should not be considered the "gold standard." Norms simply state what a tested group of people were able to do. The norms for a sit-up test performed by athletes would be considerably higher than the norms for a sit-up test performed by senior citizens. The best fitness test norms are age adjusted and based on scores from large populations. The fitness tests at the back of this book were selected with these criteria in mind. Compare yourself to these norms, but most importantly, compare yourself to yourself.

The Principle of Specificity

Would you ever practice stretching your shoulders so that you could touch your toes or do a set of curl-ups (sit-ups) to tone your legs? Of course not. You would select exercises that would accomplish your goal. When you make these selections you are using the **principle of specificity,** which states that placing a specific demand on the body results in a specific adaptation.

If you create a demand on the body by doing strength exercises, the body adapts by building stronger muscles. If you create a demand by doing aerobic exercises, the body adapts by improving the cardiorespiratory system. Note that the adaptation is specific to the demand—strength exercises result in strength, not cardiorespiratory endurance.

Different occupations place different demands on the body. As a result, ice cream scoopers have one strong arm, pianists have strong fingers, construction workers have well-developed shoulder and arm muscles, and aerobic dance instructors have toned muscles and healthy hearts. (If an occupation does create muscle imbalances, like the ice cream scooper having only one strong arm, an exercise program can often correct the imbalance.)

The Principle of Reversibility

Sometimes referred to as the **use/disuse principle,** the **principle of reversibility** is succinctly defined by the well-known phrase *use it or lose it.* Within two weeks of the time you stop exercising, your body begins to adapt to the lack of activity. The result is loss of muscle tone, flexibility, and cardiorespiratory endurance. Nobody is protected from these negative adaptations. The only way to be fit is to keep active. (Worksheet 2 will help you track your progress and stay motivated.) Varsity college athletes who stop exercising when they graduate are no better off than people who never exercised. So . . . keep moving!

The Principle of Overuse

Overuse results from violating the principle of overload. When you overdo (which is the essence of the **principle of overuse**), you create problems. Injuries, especially chronic injuries like shinsplints and tendinitis, start to appear. Some people actually become addicted to exercise. A sign of addiction is the refusal to exercise fewer than seven days a week. Addiction leads to overtraining. Signs of overtraining are the previously mentioned chronic injuries and an elevated resting heart rate. Overuse may also be the result of a violation of the principle of individuality. A person trying to keep up with another person may overload too quickly. One hundred push-ups may be an appropriate load for one individual but may be overuse for another.

SUMMARY

Your instructor has probably incorporated exercises for all five health-related fitness components into your aerobic dance exercise. Think through the class and see if you can identify at least one exercise for each fitness component.

Even though you may not know it, you are probably an expert at using the principles of exercise. For example, have you ever increased the frequency, intensity, or duration of your workout to make it more challenging? (Overload.) Have you ever asked someone for a better exercise to achieve a goal like a flatter abdomen or thinner thighs? (Specificity.) Have you ever wondered why your friend is adapting more quickly or more slowly than you are to certain parts of the class? (Individuality.) Have you ever noticed how you have more energy when you are on an exercise program than when you stop your program? (Reversibility.) Now you can consciously put these principles to work for you by creating a positive exercise plan that best fits your needs.

KNOWLEDGE TIPS

1. The five health-related fitness components are cardiorespiratory endurance, body composition, flexibility, muscular strength, and muscular endurance.

2. To overload you must go just beyond the point of comfort by increasing frequency, intensity, or time.

3. Individuals respond to exercise differently.

4. The body makes specific adaptations in accord with the demands placed upon it.

5. Deconditioning occurs with disuse.

6. Overuse results in undue fatigue, chronic injury, and other problems.

CHAPTER 3

The Aerobic Target Zone

Participants in aerobic exercise programs improve their cardiorespiratory endurance by performing within the appropriate fitness target zone. Like all target zones, the **aerobic target zone** is composed of the three variables frequency, intensity, and time (duration). In this chapter you will learn how often, how hard, and how long you must perform aerobic exercise to improve your cardiorespiratory endurance and to enjoy the associated health benefits.

Please note that this chapter is only about the target zone for aerobic exercise. The target zones for flexibility, muscular strength, and muscular endurance are described in Chapters 5 and 7.

FREQUENCY

Optimal aerobic training occurs when you exercise three to five times a week. The majority of improvement in aerobic capacity (VO_2max) occurs with three days of exercise per week. Some additional improvement may occur with four or five days of training, but the improvement starts to plateau. Exercising six or seven days a week results in little or no apparent improvement, except in weight loss. If weight loss is a primary goal, frequency can range from three to seven days a week depending on intensity, duration, and mode of exercise. Workouts of moderate intensity with longer duration and less impact are generally recommended for weight loss.

High-frequency exercisers can minimize impact stress by using low-impact, nonimpact, or nonweight-bearing activities every exercise day or on alternate days. Low-impact exercises include brisk walking and step, low-impact, and aqua (water) aerobics; nonimpact exercises include slide aerobics and some forms of aerobic dance; and nonweight-bearing exercises include swimming, rowing, cycling, and deep-water running. For a full discussion on exercise and weight loss please turn to page 107 in Chapter 11.

Exercise addicts are people who feel compelled to work out every single day. As a result, they often suffer from overuse injuries such as shinsplints and tendinitis. Some individuals develop such an obsession for exercise that they begin to value it above everything else. Like any addiction, this leads to an unhealthy lifestyle. Physical fitness must always be balanced with other wellness components such as emotional, intellectual, and spiritual health. Exercise three to five times a week and feel good about using the other two to four days to do something else.

TIME

The American College of Sports Medicine (ACSM) describes the optimal duration of a single aerobic session as 20 to 60 minutes. This range is a guideline for all aerobic activities and is not specific to aerobic dance exercise. Dr. Kenneth Cooper, director of the Institute for Aerobics Research in Dallas, Texas, recommends limiting running to 80 to 90 minutes a week at three times a week for 30 minutes or four times a week for 20 minutes. He believes that the additional benefits gained by running more (other than additional weight loss) do not outweigh the increased risk of bone, joint, and muscle injury. Since the impact stress in high-impact aerobic dance exercise is equal to or greater than that of running, the aerobic section should be limited to 20 to 30 minutes per session. If you wish to exercise aerobically for a longer duration, supplement your aerobic dance exercise with a nonimpact, low-impact, or nonweight-bearing activity.

The upper limit for activities that are less stressful to muscles and joints is 60 minutes. Exercising aerobically for more than 60 minutes brings diminishing returns. In fact, after 30 to 40 minutes, the benefits of duration, except calorie expenditure, begin to decrease. If you want to exercise longer to lose weight, you can perform activities of low to moderate intensity such as brisk walking for an hour with little worry of overuse injury. Remember, the ACSM-recommended duration for aerobic exercise is 20 to 60 minutes. However, health and fitness professionals recommend a duration of 20 to 30 minutes for high-impact aerobics since this improves cardiorespiratory endurance while minimizing the risks of overuse injury.

INTENSITY

This section contains a number of abbreviated terms. To make your reading easier, here is a quick reference list:

$$
\begin{aligned}
\text{HR} &= \text{heart rate} \\
\text{EHR} &= \text{exercise heart rate} \\
\text{RHR} &= \text{resting heart rate} \\
\text{THR} &= \text{training heart rate range} \\
&\quad \text{(target zone)} \\
\text{HRmax} &= \text{maximum heart rate} \\
\text{PreHR} &= \text{pre-exercise heart rate} \\
\text{RecHR} &= \text{recovery heart rate} \\
\text{HR}_{max}\text{reserve} &= \text{heart rate reserve } (\text{HR}_{max} - \text{RHR}) \\
\text{VO}_2\text{max} &= \text{maximum volume of oxygen} \\
&\quad \text{consumed}
\end{aligned}
$$

To comprehend how and why you monitor your workout intensity, you should understand the role of oxygen in aerobic exercise. The word *aerobic* actually means "with oxygen"; only when a steady supply of oxygen is available to the muscles can aerobic exercise be performed. The oxygen you breathe into your lungs is picked up by red blood cells and delivered to your muscles. Inside the muscle cells, oxygen is used in the chemical processes that convert food (carbohydrates, fats, and proteins) into energy for muscular contraction.

The more intensely you exercise, the more oxygen your muscles need. Your breathing becomes faster and deeper to bring in more oxygen, your heart beats faster to speed up the delivery of the oxygen, and your muscles use more food and oxygen to produce movement. As exercise becomes more and more intense, the rate and volume of oxygen entering the body continues to increase until finally the body is consuming oxygen as rapidly as it can. This maximum volume of **oxygen consumption** (measured in liters per minute or milliliters per minute per kilogram of body weight) is called **VO$_2$max;** you may also see it referred to as maximum oxygen uptake (MOU). If exercise intensity is increased any further, the muscles' demand for oxygen cannot be met. You can exercise at these very high intensities for only a short time before total exhaustion makes you stop.

Exercising at VO$_2$max is not fun. In fact, it's agonizingly difficult. The good news is that you can improve your fitness by exercising at just 50 percent of VO$_2$max. In other words, when the body's demand for oxygen is about half of what it is capable of using, aerobic conditioning begins. For this reason, 50 percent of VO$_2$max is called the **threshold of aerobic training.**

Although 50 percent of VO_2max is the threshold, cardiorespiratory fitness occurs within a range above that threshold. You should learn to stay within that range for two reasons. First, it is natural for your intensity level to fluctuate; the range lets you know how much fluctuation is acceptable. Second, you will want to target the upper or the lower end of the range depending on your fitness level. The range, according to the ACSM, is 50 to 85 percent of VO_2max.

How do you know at what percentage of VO_2max you are exercising? *You* can't count oxygen molecules. But scientists can . . . they have people ride a stationary bicycle, run on a treadmill, or use some other ergometric device while hooked up to machines that monitor oxygen consumption and heart rate. Through these laboratory tests scientists have discovered a close relationship between the number of times the heart beats per minute (**heart rate**) and the amount of oxygen a person consumes per minute. Scientists have developed two formulas based on this relationship that use heart rate instead of oxygen consumption to determine an exercise intensity range. The heart rate formulas calculate a range of acceptable heart rates—something that you can easily count by taking your **pulse,** which is the wave of pressure felt in the arteries when the heart beats.

Why two heart rate formulas instead of one? For the same reason that we measure apples in both bushels and pounds: Both are effective measures depending on the circumstances. The **maximum heart rate formula** is fairly conservative and can be calculated as long as the age of the participant is known. The **Karvonen formula** is more individualized, using both age and resting heart rate in its calculations. The resting heart rate is needed to calculate the heart rate reserve (HR_{max}reserve). Explanations for both of these formulas follow, and worksheets are available at the back of the book. Now you have enough information to understand all of the intensity ranges. According to the ACSM, the cardiorespiratory training ranges are:

50 – 85% of VO_2max (laboratory measures)

50 – 85% of HR_{max}reserve (Karvonen formula)

60 – 90% of HRmax (maximum heart rate formula)

Although a training effect occurs throughout the range, the very high intensities are significant only for competitors. As the intensity rises, so do the risk of injury and the amount of discomfort felt during the exercise. Competitive athletes have to exercise at these intensities to maintain the winning edge, but the fitness gains are not significant in relation to the risk of injury for the person interested in achieving health-related cardiorespiratory fitness.

For health-related fitness, the aerobic target zone is generally set in the middle of the cardiorespiratory training ranges previously listed. Beginners are encouraged to start at the lower values, while more fit individuals can exercise in the middle to upper parts of the following ranges:

60 – 80% of VO_2max (laboratory measures)

60 – 80% of HR_{max}reserve (Karvonen formula)

70 – 85% of HRmax (maximum heart rate formula)

Monitoring Your Intensity by Heart Rate

When the intensity range is measured by heart rate, it is called the **training heart rate range** (or target heart rate zone), usually abbreviated **THR.** To achieve aerobic conditioning you must exercise hard enough to keep your heart rate within your THR. To calculate your THR you can use either the Karvonen or the maximum heart rate formula. The Karvonen formula is more accurate, but to use it you must know your true **resting heart rate** (RHR), which is the rate at which the heart beats when the body is at rest. Although that is not difficult, it takes several days to measure. In the meantime, you may want to get started by using the quick, easy, and conservative maximum heart rate formula.

In both formulas, you will calculate a lower and an upper limit for your THR. You will need to know your **maximum heart rate** (HRmax) for both formulas. HRmax is the fastest rate your heart can beat. The most accurate way to determine your HRmax is to exercise to absolute exhaustion while your heart rate is monitored by an EKG (electrocardiograph) machine. Fortunately for you, there is a faster and easier way to determine your HRmax. Researchers discovered that the HRmax drops one beat each year of an individual's life. Through statistical extrapolation, researchers determined that a newborn's HRmax is about 220 beats per minute (bpm). A one year old would have an HRmax of 219 bpm, a two year old 218 bpm, and so on. To calculate your HRmax, simply subtract your age from 220.

220 – age (in years) = HRmax (maximum heart rate)

Maximum Heart Rate Formula (Zero to Peak Formula)

Remember, the THR is a range with an upper and a lower limit. To calculate the lower limit (threshold) of your THR, multiply your HRmax by 70 percent. To calculate the upper limit, multiply your HRmax by 85 percent. Remember that when you multiply by a percentage, you are multiplying by a fraction. For example, 70% = 70/100 = 0.70.

HRmax **x** 0.70 = lower limit of THR
HRmax **x** 0.85 = upper limit of THR

The THR for a 20-year-old person is calculated below. A space for figuring your THR is provided at the back of the book on Worksheet 3A.

Step One	Step Two	Step Three
220	200	200
−20	x .70	x .85
200	140	170
(HRmax)	(lower limit of THR)	(upper limit of THR)

Thus, the THR for this individual is 140 to 170 bpm.

Your **exercise heart rate** (EHR) is the speed at which your heart is beating during exercise. Your EHR should fall within your THR. If your EHR is higher than your THR, you are exercising too intensely. If it is lower, you aren't exercising hard enough. To find your EHR, either take your pulse while you are exercising or complete your count within 15 seconds of the time you stop. When you stop exercising, your heart rate stays at a level close to your EHR for about 15 seconds, then drops off quickly as your body recovers. During the first 15 seconds you have time to locate your pulse (most people require 2 to 4 seconds) and take a 10-second pulse count. Multiply the number of beats you count in 10 seconds by 6 to determine your pulse in beats per minute. For example,

$$\frac{25 \text{ beats}}{\cancel{10 \text{ seconds}}_{1}} \times \frac{\cancel{60 \text{ seconds}}^{6}}{1 \text{ minute}} = \frac{150 \text{ beats}}{\text{minute}}$$

Exercisers often take a 6-second count, since mentally multiplying by 10 is easy. The problem with this method is that if you miscount your heart rate, you are multiplying your error by 10. When your heart is beating very fast, it is easy to miscount by 1, even 2 beats. A 2-beat miscount becomes an error of 20 beats. If instead you use the 10-second count, a 2-beat miscount represents only a 12-beat error. Almost all fitness experts recommend the 10-second count.

To eliminate the problem of mentally multiplying by 6, convert your THR from beats per minute to beats per 10 seconds by dividing the top and bottom of the range by 6 and rounding off to the nearest whole number. The range, 140 to 170 bpm, calculated in steps one, two, and three, is converted below in steps four and five.

Step Four	Step Five	The new THR is:
$\frac{140}{6} = 23.3$	$\frac{170}{6} = 28.3$	23–28 beats/10 sec.

Looking at this example, you can see that a 20 year old who counts an EHR of 26 beats during a 10-second count is well within the recommended THR.

Karvonen Method
(Heart Rate Reserve Formula)

In this formula, percentages of the **heart rate reserve** (HR$_{max}$reserve) are calculated. The HR$_{max}$reserve is the HRmax minus the resting heart rate (RHR). The RHR is added back in after a percentage of the HR$_{max}$reserve has been calculated. The formula looks like this:

HRmax − RHR (bpm) **x** 0.60 + RHR (bpm) =
lower limit THR
HRmax − RHR (bpm) **x** 0.80 + RHR (bpm) =
upper limit THR

Before using this formula, you need an accurate count of your RHR. Take your RHR first thing in the morning while you are still lying in bed. (Relax for a few minutes if your alarm clock has jolted you into consciousness.) Count your pulse for one minute to get the rate in beats per minute. Take this RHR on two or three different mornings to determine the average rate. Individuals whose resting heart rates are influenced by disease or medication should not use the Karvonen formula.

Provided below is an example of the THR for a 20-year-old individual with an RHR of 75 bpm. To calculate your THR using the Karvonen method, turn to Worksheet 3B.

Step One	Step Four
220	75
−20	+75 (lower limit)
200 (HRmax)	150 (THR in bpm)
Step Two	Step Five
200	125
−75	x .80
125 (HR$_{max}$reserve)	100
Step Three	Step Six
125	100
x .60	+75 (upper limit)
75	175 (THR in bpm)

The range is 150 to 175 bpm (Table 3.1). Divided by six and rounded to the nearest whole number, the range is 25 to 29 beats per 10 seconds. The advantage of using the Karvonen formula is that you can adjust your THR as your RHR declines with training.

TABLE 3.1
(a) THR calculated using the Karvonen formula for a 20 year old with 75 bpm for RHR. (b) Maximum heart rate for a 20 year old with 75bpm for RHR.

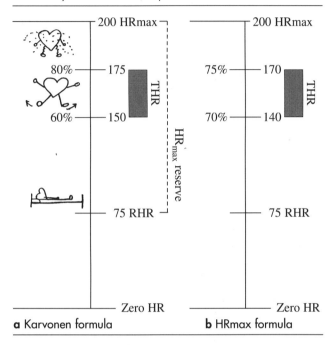

a Karvonen formula   b HRmax formula

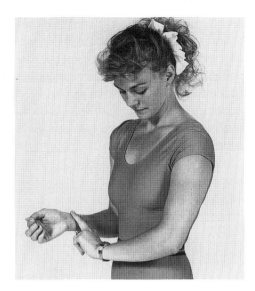

FIGURE 3.1
Radial artery.

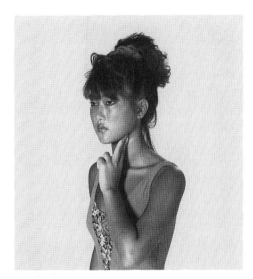

FIGURE 3.2
Carotid artery.

Taking Your Pulse

When you press gently on an **artery** you can feel the pulsing of the blood as it is pushed through the arteries by the heart. The arteries most commonly used for taking the pulse during exercise are the radial and carotid arteries.

The **radial artery** is located on the inside of your wrist. You can feel it beside your forearm tendons on the thumb side (Figure 3.1). The **carotid artery** is just to the side (either side) of your voice box (larynx). You can feel it in the valley between your Adam's apple and your neck muscles (Figure 3.2).

To feel your pulse, use two fingers to press gently but firmly on the artery. Do not use your thumb; it also has a pulse and will cause you to miscount. If you can't feel your pulse, you may be pressing too lightly or too hard. Pressing too hard on an artery squeezes it shut so that you can no longer feel any pulsing. Try different pressures while sitting quietly until you can feel and count your pulse easily. Then practice taking it while you move around the room. If you have a lot of trouble

counting your pulse, place your hand over your heart and count beats.

Although most people can use the carotid site without experiencing any problems, a word of caution is in order. Special receptors located in the walls of the carotid artery are responsible for detecting changes in pressure. If you put pressure on these baroreceptors while taking your pulse (or massage them while looking for your pulse), they send a message to the heart to slow down. This slowing heart rate can cause dizziness or faintness in some people. If your heart rate does slow down, your pulse count will not be accurate. Try taking your pulse at both your carotid and your radial sites. If you find the carotid gives you a slower count, use the radial site.

When taking your pulse, count complete cardiac cycles. A pulse throb constitutes the end of a cardiac cycle. If the instructor says *go* and you immediately feel a throb, don't count it (or call it zero). If the instructor says *go* and there is a pause and then a beat, go ahead and count it as number one. Continue to count until the instructor stops you.

Other Heart Rates

Other heart rates in addition to the EHR are useful to monitor and compare. For example, the resting heart rate is also a useful indicator of cardiorespiratory fitness. As your fitness improves, your heart becomes stronger and your circulatory system more efficient. This means that your heart can beat fewer times per minute and still accomplish the same amount of work. Think of how many times you have to work the handle on an inefficient pump to get a gallon of water compared to the number of times you have to work the handle on an efficient pump. Your heart acts like a pump. As your heart and circulatory system improve, you will be able to see a decline in your resting heart rate. Remember the principle of individuality; some people's RHRs will decline quickly and dramatically, while those of others will hardly decline at all. An average RHR is 70 to 80 bpm. Highly trained athletes often have RHRs as low as 45, but some elite runners have RHRs in the 60s and 70s. (These athletes were highly efficient in some other physiological way.) Take your RHR periodically to see if it is declining.

Besides heredity and exercise, a number of other factors influence the RHR. Medication, illness, stress, overtraining, temperature, caffeine, and smoking are a few of the major influences. Since many of these influences are transient, you probably won't pick them up in a morning resting heart rate. They will, however, often show up in a heart rate taken right before class. For example, your **pre-exercise heart rate** (PreHR) can be elevated if you are still digesting a meal, just drank a cup of caffeinated coffee or a can of soda, ran to class, or are anxious about a test in the next class. Take your PreHR before you begin exercising, plot it on the chart provided in Worksheet 4, and see if you can identify reasons for any fluctuations you discover.

Another useful heart rate to monitor is your **recovery heart rate** (RecHR), which reflects the speed with which your cardiorespiratory system can return to its pre-exercise state after you stop exercising. It is often used as an indicator of fitness because a physically fit person with an efficient cardiorespiratory system generally recovers from exercise more quickly than an unfit person exercising at the same intensity. The heart rate drops rapidly during the first minute of recovery, then more slowly and gradually drops to normal. Many people are able to return to a heart rate below 120 bpm within two minutes. If you are not below 120 bpm in five minutes, your THR is probably too high for your fitness level. (You may also have performed too active a cooldown.) Continue to cool down until your pulse is below 120 bpm.

To monitor your RecHR, take your pulse immediately after the aerobic portion of class and again one minute later. Record your RecHR on the chart provided in Worksheet 4. Your instructor may wish to use a two-, three-, or five-minute recovery time instead of a one-minute time. Any recovery time will work as long as you are consistent, although more fit people may want to use the shorter times since most of their recovery will occur in the first two minutes. You should see an improved recovery rate after about 6 to 12 weeks of aerobic conditioning.

Keeping track of these heart rates can make you more aware of the kinds of things (exercise, stress, caffeine, and others) that affect your body. Table 3.2 is an example of a heart rate chart in progress for a 20-year-old individual. The THR is drawn in bold lines. The PreHR, EHR, and RecHR have been recorded for each exercise session. Lines connecting the same types of heart rates have been drawn to make it easier to see the trends. Some trends to look for include a more consistent EHR with practice, a lower RecHR over time, and an increased ability to work in the upper portion of the THR.

Alternative Methods of Calculating and Monitoring Intensity

A Swedish physiologist named Gunnar Borg discovered a relationship between the perception of exercise intensity and heart rate. He developed the **rating of perceived exertion** (RPE) scale shown in Table 3.3. To use this scale, look at the numbers and word descriptions and select the number that best represents how hard you feel (perceive) you are exercising. Perceived exertion ratings between 12 and 18 produce a training effect. Research evidence indicates that the RPE scale is an effective way for adults to monitor aerobic intensity.

When first using the RPE scale, it is a good idea to make ratings and then check heart rate. When you know which ratings coincide best with your target heart rate range and are consistently labeling the same heart rate

TABLE 3.2
Heart rate chart in progress.

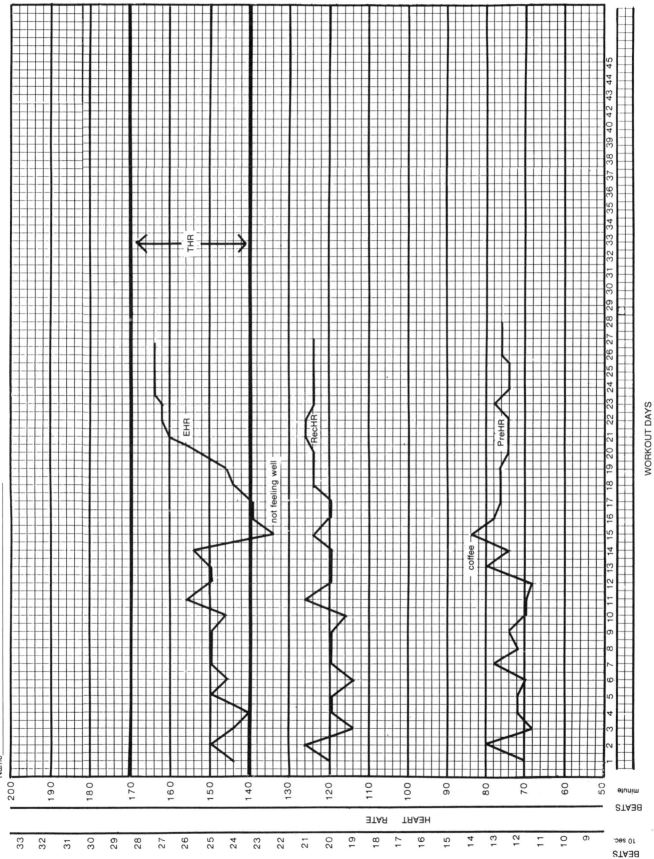

TABLE 3.3
Rating of perceived exertion (RPE) scale.

6.	
7.	Very, very light
8.	
9.	Very light
10.	
11.	Fairly light
12.	
13.	Somewhat hard
14.	
15.	Hard
16.	
17.	Very hard
18.	
19.	Very, very hard
20.	

From: G. V. Borg, *Medicine and Science in Sports and Exercise* 14 (1982): 377–87.

with the same RPE, you can start to phase out taking your pulse and rely more on ratings of perceived exertion. In essence what you are doing is learning how to listen to your body so you can know how hard you are working.

RPE also works when heart rate is not reliable. If, for example, you are on a medication that affects heart rate, or if you aren't good at taking a pulse count, RPE can be a good method for estimating workout intensity.

Another quick, easy (and less scientific) method for estimating intensity is the talk test. You should be able to talk comfortably while working out. If you can't, your workout intensity is too high. If you can sing comfortably, your intensity is probably too low.

When to Monitor Intensity

Using the pulse check, the RPE scale, or the talk test, you should monitor your level of exertion periodically during your workout. It is a good idea to check your intensity level 5 to 10 minutes into the aerobic workout to make sure you have reached your training intensity. Check again at the peak of the aerobic section to make sure you aren't too high. Check once again toward the end of the aerobic section to see whether you were able to maintain the training intensity to the end. If you check your intensity only at the end of class and find that you are too high or too low, it is too late to modify your workout. In addition, your finishing heart rate may not be indicative of the intensity of your entire workout.

Exercise Levels

Individuals who have not been exercising regularly, who are returning to exercise after an injury, or who are substantially overweight (overfat) should start exercising at the low end of the target zone. For some beginners, even threshold amounts of exercise may be too much of an overload. In this event, start with small, manageable workout segments, 3–10 minutes long. Start with walking, cycling, swimming, or easy dance steps and work up to more formal aerobic dance exercises. To overload, first increase the frequency of the short bouts and then start to increase duration by putting short bouts together. When you can perform for 20–30 minutes, overload by increasing intensity. If burning fat is your goal, increase duration to 30–60 minutes (depending on the activity), maintaining a moderate intensity.

As you become more fit you will find that you have to use more arm work and larger ranges of motion to challenge your aerobic system. Big movements are recommended, but avoid the use of momentum and do not overextend the limits of your flexibility.

Research has shown that aerobic dance activity results in cardiorespiratory training similar to that of jogging and cycling. However, physiologists have not yet determined whether aerobic dance activity can train and maintain very high fitness levels. If you are interested in a competitive level of aerobic conditioning, you may have to combine aerobic dance training with other forms of aerobic exercise. I have had a few highly fit runners in my classes who, even with vigorous movement, were unable to reach the upper ranges of their THR. These individuals used aerobic dance exercise for light workout days and change of pace, while everyone else worked up a heavy sweat! Step aerobics, particularly with power moves, may be able to challenge even the most fit. Advanced participants, give it a try!

SUMMARY

To improve your aerobic fitness you must exercise above your aerobic threshold and within your aerobic target zone. The target zone is described by the FIT variables: frequency, intensity, and time. Optimum cardiorespiratory fitness occurs when you exercise three to five times a week, at 50 to 85 percent of heart rate reserve, for 20 to 60 minutes. When aerobic dance exercise is the mode of training, the duration of the aerobic routines should be shortened to 20 to 30 minutes and performed at an intensity of 60 to 80 percent of heart rate reserve. This level of exercise will promote health and minimize overuse injuries. Beginners should start out near their threshold levels of frequency, intensity, and time. That means exercising three times a week for 20 minutes at an intensity equal to 50 percent of HR_{max}reserve. When beginners need to start out below threshold, they should first gradually increase time and frequency and then intensity. Advanced participants can, of course, work out at the higher end of their ranges.

KNOWLEDGE TIPS

1. Participants can monitor the intensity of an aerobic workout using pulse counts, ratings of perceived exertion, or the talk test.

2. The pulse should be counted for 10 seconds using the radial or carotid site.

3. Participants should monitor their intensity several times during the workout to make sure they are working in their aerobic target zone.

4. The best measures of oxygen consumption and maximum heart rate are obtained through direct measurement during a graded exercise stress test (on a treadmill or stationary bicycle). From these measures an accurate THR can be calculated.

5. Formulas have been derived to estimate the THR without direct measures of oxygen consumption and maximum heart rate.

6. The Karvonen formula calculates THRs very similar to those obtained in graded exercise tests. To use this formula you must first obtain an accurate reading of your resting heart rate; 60 to 80 percent of the HR_{max}reserve is calculated.

7. The maximum heart rate formula underestimates the THR by about 15 percent. To compensate, 70 to 85 percent of the HRmax is used instead of the 60 to 80 percent range used with the Karvonen formula.

8. Training below threshold may produce fitness gains for individuals at very low fitness levels.

9. The resting heart rate and recovery heart rate can also be used as indicators of fitness.

CHAPTER 4

Setting Goals and Reaching Your Dream

Do you dream of looking svelte, sporting beautifully toned muscles, living longer, and feeling radiantly full of energy? Then act on that dream by embarking on a sensible exercise program that includes specific and realistic goals.

Millions of people enroll in exercise classes, buy fancy outfits and equipment, and talk enthusiastically about the fun and benefits, but within six months of the time they started, 30 to 70 percent of these people drop out. Even many former varsity athletes and coaches who have spent most of their lives promoting fitness are overweight (overfat) and out of shape. Ironically, the majority of people, even nonexercisers, have a good attitude about exercise.

Why then do so many people quit or never get started? Physical educators, fitness specialists, and exercise scientists have been trying to answer that question. What they have learned through research and observation can be synthesized to form a positive plan of action for adherence.

First, establish clear, precise, specific, measurable goals. Second, find and use sources of motivation. Third, select an activity (or activities), such as aerobic dance exercise, that will help you reach your goals. Fourth, establish a method for measuring progress. Finally, establish a process for evaluating your goals and your program to make sure they are what you want and need and that they are functioning properly. Each of these steps is explained more thoroughly in this chapter.

STEP ONE: ESTABLISHING YOUR FITNESS GOALS

The Basis for Your Goals

A goal is a statement of what you want to happen. Base your fitness goals on what you would like to accomplish through an exercise program. Write down any ideas that come to mind. For example, you might create a list like the following: lose weight, lose inches, be able to touch toes, walk up the stairs without getting tired, or run five miles. In addition to basing your goals on personal desire, you can use the five health-related fitness components as guidelines. Try to think of at least one goal for each fitness component: cardiorespiratory endurance, flexibility, body composition, muscular strength, and muscular endurance.

Guidelines in this chapter, information in other parts of this book, fitness test scores, and guidance from your instructor will help you to refine the goals you have identified and to select goals you may not have considered. Base your goals on personal interest (desire), fitness test results, and knowledge of what is realistic, feasible, and healthy.

This chapter focuses on physical fitness goals. Some very valuable goals cannot be measured by fitness tests or, in some cases, be adequately tested for at all. Your list might also include some of these goals, such as increased social involvement, improvement of self-concept, improvement of self-confidence, achievement of relaxation, and having fun. You can often measure progress toward goals such as these by keeping a journal. For example, if your goal is to have more energy so you can be more productive, then keeping a journal that tracks your accomplishments and how you feel at the end of a day will give you an idea of how you are progressing.

Specific Goals

When asked to write down their goals for the semester, the majority of my college students write things such as:

· Lose weight

· Lose inches

· Last longer in the class

· Look better

· Become more fit

· Firm up my body

The ideas expressed provide a starting point, but they are ambiguous; students have no concrete way to measure success. For example, does the loss of one pound constitute success? Does looking better mean an attractive appearance or how you look doing the exercises? Does lasting longer mean during the body toning exercises, aerobic exercises, or both? At what point is the body firm?

These goals can be rewritten to be more specific. They might read like this:

· Lose 10 pounds in the next 10 weeks (a safe 1-pound loss per week)

· Lose 1 inch from each thigh, my waist, and my hips by the end of the semester

· Complete 20 minutes of standing aerobics at 70 to 85 percent of my maximum heart rate

· Tone and firm my legs as represented by losing 1 inch from my thighs and being able to do 25 percent more leg lifts in a row

· Complete the 3 minutes of the step test

· Increase my 1-minute sit-up score from a poor rating to an average rating

These very specific goals can be measured, full or partial success can be noted and celebrated, and new goals can be set.

Realistic Goals

Beginners and overzealous participants have a tendency to choose unrealistic goals. When you set goals that are too difficult, you set yourself up for failure. Yet, goals that are too easy aren't very motivating. Three guidelines for writing challenging and yet attainable goals are (1) allow enough time to reach the goal, (2) set safe goals, and (3) base goals on correct information.

1. Positive adaptations do not occur overnight. It usually takes six to eight weeks to make significant cardiorespiratory and muscular gains. It can take longer to strengthen ligaments, bones, and tendons. Be patient and write your goals with time expectations of at least six to eight weeks. People who expect quick results often quit the program before it has had a chance to work. Start with conservative goals so you have success early in the program.

2. To set safe goals, consider your medical history, your present condition, your age, and the amount of

time that has passed since you last exercised. Set up a pace and program that are comfortable for you. There is no need to start out too fast and get stiff, sore, or injured. The idea is to have fun and feel good about exercising.

Many unsafe goals arise from the desire to obtain quick results. For example, people who want very rapid weight loss starve themselves and at the same time attempt to attend an exercise class. Without a sufficient intake of carbohydrates they don't have enough energy to exercise. They may feel listless, tired, dizzy, or even faint during class. Starvation diets result in significant loss of muscle and water, not just fat. The body may even start conserving and storing fat as an energy source because the caloric intake is so low.

3. Misconceptions can wreak havoc on goals. For example, a person with a goal of losing abdominal fat might embark on an intense program of curl-ups. When he or she can do 100 curl-ups a day and finds the fat still there, discouragement is sure to set in. The problem is that fat is lost through aerobic exercise, not anaerobic exercise such as curl-ups. The result of doing curl-ups will be strong abdominal muscles hiding under a layer of fat. In addition, fat cannot be taken off in one specific spot (spot reduction); it comes off in a general way from all over the body.

Faulty reasoning can also be dangerous. There have been cases of pregnant women whose reason for exercising during pregnancy was to keep their figures. These women were trying to prevent normal weight gains, and if allowed to continue, they would endanger the health of their babies. Pregnant women can benefit from exercise as long as it is done correctly and with the supervision of a doctor.

The best way to avoid making these kinds of mistakes is to read about fitness from reliable sources (books and articles written by professionals and materials published by recognized associations such as the American College of Sports Medicine, the American College of Obstetricians and Gynecologists, and the American Alliance for Health, Physical Education, Recreation, and Dance) and to talk with professionals like your instructor.

It is also important to remember the principle of individuality as you try to set realistic goals. Two people on an identical exercise program will respond differently. It can be motivating to compare yourself against norms or averages or even classmates, but remember, the comparison that counts is you against you.

Short- and Long-Range Goals

Take your dream, your long-range goal, and break it down into short-range goals. If your dream is to lose three inches off your waist, make short-term goals of one-half inch every eight weeks. Reaching the short-term goal will give you the confidence and motivation to keep going. One step at a time will take you to your dream.

When you don't make short-term goals, you set yourself up for total success or total failure: There is nothing in between. If reaching your goal takes a while and you have no intermediate steps of success to celebrate, it is easy to get discouraged and quit. Think of the people who climb Mt. Everest: They are pleased when they establish base camp, and they cheer as they establish each successive camp up the mountain. Their goal is the summit, but they recognize that success comes in stages.

Fitness professionals can help you set realistic specific goals, tell you what a realistic rate of achievement is, provide encouragement, and evaluate and adjust your program. These people are service oriented and want to help you. They are your instructor, physical educators in your schools, service coordinators, directors in fitness clubs, owners and directors of private fitness businesses, professors and instructors at colleges and universities, and instructors and coordinators at recreation centers, YMCAs, and corporate programs. Seek them out.

STEP TWO: FINDING MOTIVATION

People usually start exercising to look good, but the main reason habitual exercisers give for continuing is that exercise feels good. Endorphins, hormonelike substances, are released during exercise; scientists believe that in addition to masking pain, endorphins are responsible for the uplifting feeling that follows a good workout. Unfortunately, many people just starting out have never felt this exercise "high" and can't identify with it. And since it takes six to eight weeks to work into the exercise high, many quit before they experience this wonderful benefit.

In the beginning, you may feel a little stiff, sore, and awkward. The trick is to get past this discomfort so that you can experience the good feelings that come from exercise. Once you do experience the exercise high, often accompanied by an increased sense of energy, you'll find it motivates you to keep on exercising.

There are two forms of motivation: intrinsic and extrinsic. **Intrinsic motivation** comes from inside you. If you exercise because you want to look and feel better, then you are intrinsically motivated. **Extrinsic motivation** comes from outside you. It may be in the form of a television commercial selling soda and fitness, a spouse offering you a lobster dinner if you exercise for three months, or a friend calling you up to see if you'll be in class today.

When you personally believe in something, you will be more motivated to do it than if someone else is telling you to do it. Find an exercise program that is taught in a style that you like, at a place you enjoy, and at a time and in a location that is convenient for you—aspects that are intrinsically motivating. If you do this, you will be more likely to stick with your program.

You may be one of those rare and wonderful people who have the internal desire and discipline to exercise all of their life. If so, fantastic! But if you are like most of us and need the proverbial "kick in the pants" to keep motivated, here are a few sources of extrinsic motivation you can tap:

1. Find another person who also wants to exercise and make a pact to meet at a designated place on workout days. Knowing that other person is waiting for you will get you there. Car pools with rotating drivers also provide an extra incentive to show up, especially if you are the driver.

2. Get the people around you—friends, family, and fellow employees—to support or join you in your exercise endeavors. Plan family outings that involve hiking, swimming, cycling, and other forms of exercise. Organize a college or corporate team to participate in a local road race or aerobithon. Nothing is worse than having someone resent you for taking an hour out of your day to exercise. Try to get them interested too.

3. Find sources of feedback and reinforcement. Get to know your instructor and find out if you are doing things correctly. A good instructor will be complimentary, will provide feedback periodically, and will miss you when you are not there. It is much more difficult to miss a class when the instructor or participants are going to give you a hard time for not being there. Some really ambitious instructors even call to find out what has happened to you when you miss two classes in a row.

4. Write down your goals and look at them periodically. Some people like to post their goals on their bathroom mirror or refrigerator door so they will see them often. Perhaps it will help you to tell someone about your goals, especially if that person is in a position to help you attain them. For example, your instructor may be able to introduce you to someone else with the same goal.

5. Set aside a specific time for your exercise and don't let anything but an emergency interfere with it.

6. Do something nice for yourself and others when you reach a short-term goal.

7. Finally, accept that you will have lapses. We are all human. Illness, emergencies, vacation, or even boredom can take you temporarily off your program. It doesn't mean that you are a miserable failure. Just pick a date to begin again and go forth with new resolve.

STEP THREE: CHOOSING THE ACTIVITY

If your goal is to be aerobically fit, you have a wide variety of activities from which to choose: walking, swimming, cycling, rowing, cross-country skiing, stair stepping, jumping rope, aerobic dancing and many others. Select an activity you enjoy. For the sake of this book, let's assume you've decided on aerobic dance exercise.

If, however, for some reason you begin to lose interest in aerobic dance exercise, it starts to hurt your knees, or for whatever reason you find it doesn't suit you, please do not give up exercising; select a new activity. Do something you enjoy, and you will stay at it much longer.

STEP FOUR: MEASURING YOUR PROGRESS

To measure progress you must have a starting point; a good one is your present fitness level. You can measure it using one of the many fitness tests that have been developed over the years. The ones contained in this text were selected because of their relationship to the health-related fitness components. Table 4.1 is a list of these tests under their appropriate fitness component heading. Each test is described in detail on the designated worksheet provided at the back of the book or in the appropriate chapter. The norms provided with these tests should give you a general idea of how well you scored.

Don't be too concerned with the norms; it is more important to compare your scores at the beginning of a program to your scores later in the program.

TABLE 4.1
Fitness tests.

Cardiorespiratory Endurance Tests	
1. Step Tests	Worksheets 5A, 5B
2. 12-Minute Walk/Run	Worksheet 5C
3. 1.5-Mile Run	Worksheet 5D
Flexibility	
1. Sit-and-Reach Test	Worksheet 6A
2. Five Pass/Fail Flexibility Tests	Worksheet 6B
Muscular Strength and Endurance	
1. Curl-Up Tests	Worksheet 7A
2. Push-Up Test	Worksheet 7B
Body Composition	
1. Skin-Fold Technique	Chapter 11
2. Underwater Weighing	Chapter 11
3. Impedance Technique	Chapter 11

Some fitness tests can be taken right at the beginning of a program. Other, more difficult tests, such as the 12-minute walk/run test and the 1.5-mile timed run test, should be taken only after you've been exercising for about 6 weeks. Retake the tests after about 8 to 12 weeks to see how you are progressing. It is very motivating to see tangible evidence of improvement. (You may even see improvement in 6 weeks, but don't be discouraged if you see no improvement.) You may discover that you are very fit in one component and not so fit in another. Follow a program that lets you maintain your strengths and improve your weaknesses.

STEP FIVE: EVALUATING THE PROGRAM AND YOUR GOALS

After you have been exercising for 6 to 8 weeks, it is important to take an objective look at your program to see if it is accomplishing what you intended. Look at your goals and the results of your most recent set of fitness test scores. If your goals also included things such as meeting new people, ask yourself how many new friends you have made. If the results of your program don't indicate achievement toward your goals, something is wrong; change the goals, or change the program.

Sometimes goals change. For example, teenagers often base their goals on a desire to have an incredible body while adults place more emphasis on weight control and a healthy body. As retirement approaches, people tend to shift their goals again, this time toward sociability and maintaining physical independence. Keep your goals up-to-date and adjust your program whenever your goals change.

Sometimes you don't follow your own exercise plan. This can happen if the instructor and class have a plan different from yours, if you get injured and have to modify your plan, if you don't like part of the plan and decide not to do it, or if you don't have enough time to work at your whole plan. When these things happen, reassess your priorities and try to create a new plan of attack.

If the class you are in is different from what you expected and you cannot change classes, see if the instructor will let you individualize your workout enough to satisfy you both. For example, if you really want to develop strong abdominal muscles and the class emphasis is on leg work, see if you can do some abdominal exercises while the class continues with leg work.

When you aren't doing something because you dislike it, see if another exercise can accomplish the same thing. For instance, some people don't like or can't do push-ups. An arm-pushing exercise using an exercise band can be substituted. If no substitutes are practical, you must decide whether an exercise is vital enough to your health that you should do it even though you don't like it.

In the event of injury, extend the time period on your goal and be patient. If you don't have enough time to work on your entire plan, determine your highest priorities and put time where you need it most.

Sometimes your personal exercise program isn't working. You may be using insufficient overloads or the wrong exercises. Check with your instructor and redesign your program.

In other cases, the program is working, but it is not reflected in the goals. Take, for example, a person whose goal is to lose weight. Eight weeks of aerobics later, she is discouraged because she has gained weight. Upon closer examination, however, she discovers that she has lost inches and has a lower percentage of body fat; she actually lost fat and gained muscle. Since muscle weighs more than fat, she gained weight. The program worked, but the goal didn't reflect the improvement.

Sometimes, a new and better exercise program comes along. If you hear of a new program, find out if it is based on solid information and backed by people with good credentials. Exercise research generates new information, resulting in new and sometimes better program ideas. For example, 30 years ago it was thought that weight training would inhibit strength. Football players were not allowed to lift weights! Today we know that weight training is a good way to improve muscular strength, and it is being incorporated into aerobic dance exercise through the use of hand and ankle weights and exercise bands. Be open-minded when it comes to new ideas, but beware of promises of instant success.

SUMMARY

With the help of your instructor, determine your fitness goals and set up a plan of action. Make the plan specific and realistic, then stick with it. Check your progress and celebrate improvement. Update your fitness plan throughout your life, and it will continue to bring you satisfaction and joy.

KNOWLEDGE TIPS

1. The dropout rate in exercise programs is between 30 and 70 percent within six months of beginning the program. Certain strategies may improve adherence.

2. Goals are based on personal desires, fitness test scores, information from knowledgeable sources, and advice from professional educators.

3. Establish clear, precise, specific, and (whenever possible) measurable goals.

4. For motivational purposes, break long-range goals into a series of short-range goals.

5. Intrinsic motivation comes from within yourself and is the most powerful form of motivation. Extrinsic motivation comes from outside sources. Use both.

6. Select exercise activities that will help you reach your goals. Vary these activities as needed.

7. Use fitness tests to measure your current fitness levels and continue to check your progress using the same tests.

8. Periodically evaluate your exercise goals and programs to make sure that they are up-to-date and complement each other.

CHAPTER 5

Warming Up and Cooling Down

WARM-UP

The purpose of the **warm-up** is to prepare your body for activity. Many people come to an aerobic dance–exercise class after being sedentary most of the day. Muscles tight from sitting in class, working at a desk, bending over machinery, or sitting in a car need to be awakened, warmed up, and stretched out. If you exercise early in the morning, the warm-up is even more important since your muscles have been inactive all night.

First, you literally need to make your body warm. Easy, active movements to energizing music start the blood circulating and raise the body's core temperature. This is called the core warm-up. The second part of the warm-up consists of stretching exercises. It takes about 5 to 10 minutes to prepare the body for action.

Core Warm-Up Technique

It is critical that warm-up activity start out slow and easy and then build to a moderate pace. This pace allows muscles to warm and become elastic. Warm muscles are capable of more forceful, rapid movements and are less vulnerable to injury. Starting slowly also gives the cardiorespiratory system a chance to adjust gradually to the increasing oxygen demand of the muscles. Sudden vigorous activity is hard on your body, and the shunting of blood to the muscles may leave you light-headed. Just think how you feel right after you sprint to board the subway just before the door closes or jump out of the way of danger. To prevent this jarring feeling start gradually and give your heart and muscles a chance to adjust.

Warm-up activity also signals the secretion of synovial fluid. This fluid, secreted into the joints, acts as a lubricant. Much like the tin man in the *Wizard of Oz,* you need to "oil up" your joints. Start out with small movements, and as the joints and muscles respond, work up to bigger ones.

The warm-up is a good time to mentally prepare yourself for exercise. Set aside the worries of the day and release yourself to a fun-filled hour of invigorating exercise. Concentrate on the following four technique tips during the core warm-up:

1. Begin the class with easy movements. Use exercises that require a normal range of motion rather than excessive flexibility. You won't want to put a lot of stretch and pull on your muscles until they are warm. For example, reaching one arm up overhead and then the other is good, but stretching your arm way up and as far across the body as possible is too much. Walking, light jogging, easy dance steps, and light arm work are all good warm-up activities.

2. Start with small movements and work up to bigger ones. For example, start a shoulder warm-up by just lifting and rotating your shoulders while your arms hang relaxed at your sides. Next do a circling motion with your arms, letting your elbows draw the circle. Last, work the circles with straight, but not locked, arms.

3. Work with smooth movements. This is not a time for bouncing or jarring your muscles and joints. Use flowing, sustained movements, and allow your body to make the transition from a sedentary day to an active class.

4. Move at a moderate pace. You want to move vigorously enough to raise your core temperature and activate the synovial fluid, which lubricates your joints, but not so fast that momentum carries your limbs beyond a comfortable range of motion.

Warm-Up Stretch Technique

Cold muscles are like cold taffy—a quick pull and they snap. Warm taffy stretches and stretches. So, warm up your muscles first and then stretch them. The warm-up stretch is designed to prepare your muscles for action and prevent injury. The cool-down stretch, when your muscles are really warm, is the time to work on developing more flexibility.

Experts agree that you should stretch following activity, but they do not all agree that stretching before an activity is valuable. More research needs to be done in this area. It has been my experience that people feel more ready for exercise after stretching. Also, older individuals may need more prestretching than younger individuals. Most instructors provide a prestretch either after the core warm-up or in combination with it.

Flexibility is the range of movement you have around a joint. Sometimes this flexibility is taken for granted, and it's not until you lose flexibility that you realize how much it affects your daily life. Just think how much flexibility is required to raise your arms to take off a shirt, to throw a ball, or to do the tango. These movements are effortless when you have good range of motion, painfully difficult when you don't. To appreciate flexibility, imagine that you have a stiff neck and try to go a few hours without turning your head independently of your body.

As you get older, your independence is, to a large degree, dependent on your flexibility. (I recently cringed while I watched one of my older relatives try, and fail, to bend over far enough to pick up her purse from the floor.) Regardless of your age, you can always improve your flexibility. However, it is much easier to develop and maintain flexibility when you are young than to start to develop it when you are older.

When stretching a muscle, move slowly into the stretch position and then hold for a minimum of 10 seconds. Stretch to a point of discomfort but not to pain. Pain is your body's way of saying that something is wrong. If you feel pain during a stretch, back off a little or relax the muscle and start over.

Holding a stretch position (**static stretching**) convinces the muscle that it should lengthen. If you bounce (or pulse) while stretching, the muscle is put rapidly in and out of a stretch position: this is called **ballistic stretching.** Located in the muscle tissue are special sensors that keep track of muscle tension. If a muscle is suddenly stretched, the sensors fire off a message to tighten the muscle so that it won't be overstretched, damaged, or torn from the bone. Ballistic stretching alerts this protective mechanism, resulting in some muscle tightening—the opposite of the effect desired in a stretch. Static stretching is more gentle and does not alert these sensors and is therefore the preferred way of stretching.

Ballistic stretching is not, however, without merit. Once you have warmed up and statically stretched, ballistic stretching or ballistic warm-up movements can help prepare you for an activity that will use quick or explosive movements. The important thing is to precede ballistic stretches with static stretches and to use static stretches at the end of the workout to promote flexibility.

The flexibility target zone is described by the three variables frequency, intensity, and time. To improve flexibility, stretch three to seven days a week and hold each stretch for at least 10 seconds. For optimal development of flexibility, hold stretches for 20 to 60 seconds. Repeat the stretches one to three times. One 30-second hold is usually more effective than three 10-second holds. The intensity is best described by stretching to a point of discomfort but not pain.

You may want to build several different methods of stretching into your workout. Each method facilitates stretching in a different way. In **assisted** or **passive stretching,** a partner holds you in a stretch. While the partner does the holding, you can relax and let the muscle lengthen. Assisted stretching works very well when you have a trustworthy partner. **Antagonist stretching** works on the principle that when one muscle is contracted, its paired muscle is lengthened (stretched). The contracted muscle is the **agonist;** the relaxed muscle is the **antagonist.** During a stretch exercise you can help relax a muscle by consciously contracting its paired muscle. In **PNF (proprioceptive neuromuscular facilitation) stretching,** you perform an isometric contraction for 6 to 10 seconds first, then relax the muscle and stretch it. A reflex action helps relax the muscle so that it can be stretched. PNF stretching is most often used for rehabilitation. The mechanisms behind PNF and antagonist stretching are explained more fully in Chapter 10.

If you have been physically inactive during the day, it is important to start your workout gently. Women who wear high heels keep their Achilles tendon in a shortened position all day. The transition from high heels to flat-soled aerobic shoes must be made carefully. Too often, people who are late to class skip the warm-up and jump directly into vigorous activity. This is a good way to aggravate your Achilles tendon, other muscles, and your cardiorespiratory system. If you are late to class, please start slowly, warm up, and stretch the important muscle groups.

The following is a series of stretches for the body's major muscle groups. Only the major muscles being stretched are labeled; however, a number of smaller muscles will also be stretched during these exercises. The stretches are described for one side only (the side pictured), but they should be done on both sides. Emphasis is placed on body alignment. During any stretches performed in a standing position, be sure to hold the abdominal region in, the back and pelvis straight, and the knees slightly bent.

NECK STRETCHES
Muscles stretched: neck flexors, extensors

1. Rotating or holding the head to the sides and front provides a nice stretch of the neck muscles (Figures 5.1a, 5.1b, 5.1c). Rolling or laying the head to the back places pressure on the cervical vertebrae. Avoiding this position is probably healthier over the long run. If you are warming up for a sport activity that requires the head to drop backward, such as gymnastics, wrestling, or football, then it is a good idea to stretch to the back. Since aerobics does not require the head to drop backward, there is no reason to place stress on the vertebrae.

   Variation to exercise 5.1a Lifting the chin after fully rotating the head adds a little extra stretch to the neck muscles.

2. Perform neck glides by pulling in the chin as though you are trying to create a double chin (Figure 5.2). Hold for two to three seconds and release. Do 5–10 neck glides. This exercise helps counter the tendency to let the chin protrude and can be performed any time during the day when neck fatigue is experienced.

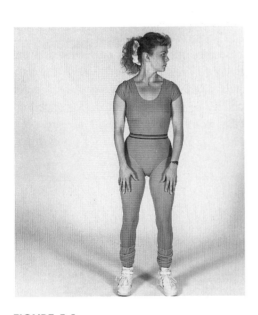

FIGURE 5.1a

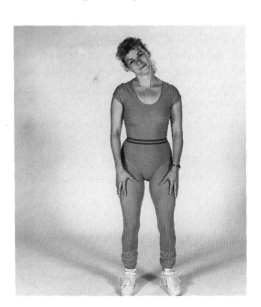

FIGURE 5.1b

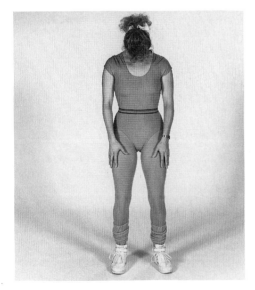

FIGURE 5.1c

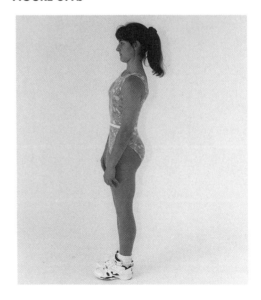

FIGURE 5.2

SHOULDER STRETCHES
Muscles stretched: deltoids, triceps, pectorals

1. Stretch the left arm across the front of the body parallel to the floor. Place the right hand above the left elbow and gently apply pressure across and in toward the chest (Figure 5.3).

2. Reach the right arm straight up. Bend at the elbow and try to touch the right hand to the middle of the back. Place the left hand just above the right elbow and push the arm into a stretch position (Figure 5.4). Drop the head forward slightly for comfort.

3. Grasp the hands behind the back, interlacing the fingers. Try to raise the arms upward. Bend forward slightly at the waist with the knees bent (Figure 5.5).

4. Lift arms out to the sides with palms facing front. Have a partner very gently and smoothly pull the arms backward (Figure 5.6). Be sure the partner grasps the arms between elbows and shoulders, so that pressure on the elbow joint is avoided.

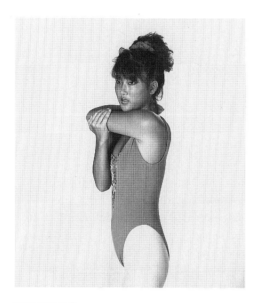

FIGURE 5.3

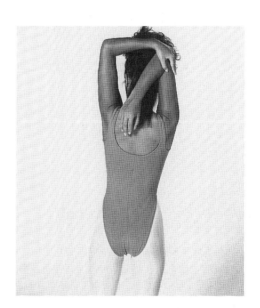

FIGURE 5.4

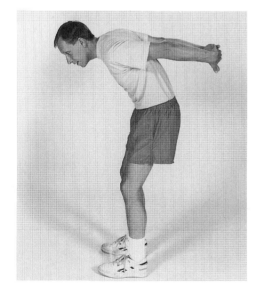

FIGURE 5.5

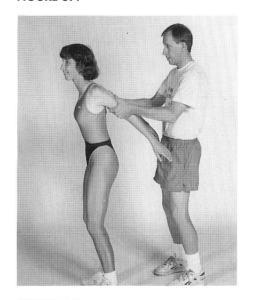

FIGURE 5.6

BACK STRETCH

Muscles stretched: erector spinae, other back muscles

Stand with feet shoulder width apart and knees bent. Tuck the pelvis under by contracting the abdomen. Grasp the hands in front of the body with palms facing outward. Try to cave in or hollow out the chest and abdominal areas (Figure 5.7). The back should appear rounded. Allow the head to follow the natural line of the curve.

Variation You can also perform this exercise with the hands on the knees, rounding and then relaxing the back.

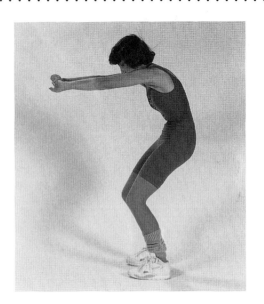

FIGURE 5.7

SIDE STRETCH

Muscles stretched: obliques, intercostals

Place the feet shoulder width apart. If stretching to the right, be sure that the right foot is angled outward and the right knee is bent. This keeps the torso, knee, and foot all going in the same direction and decreases the chance of knee soreness. Bend directly to the right side. The left arm can be relaxed by your side or extended for balance (Figure 5.8a) or, for a more advanced stretch, extended up by the left ear (Figure 5.8b). For added support, place the right hand on the thigh of the bent right leg.

If this position is held for an extended amount of time, pressure is put on the vertebral discs. Controlled movement into and out of the position is recommended.

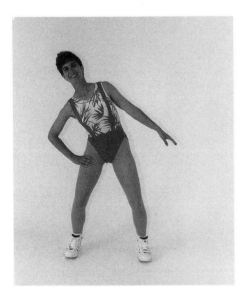

FIGURE 5.8a

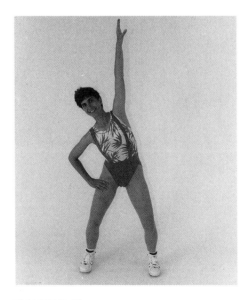

FIGURE 5.8b

BUTTOCKS STRETCHES
Muscles stretched: gluteals

1. Lie on the floor on your back with knees bent. Place the right foot on the left knee. Grasp the left

thigh and gently pull the left thigh toward the chest (Figure 5.9).

2. Kneel down with the hands on the floor close to the knees. Lean over to one side until you feel a stretch in the buttocks muscles on that side (Figure 5.10). If this hurts the knees, use a different stretch.

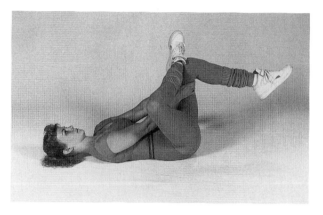

FIGURE 5.9

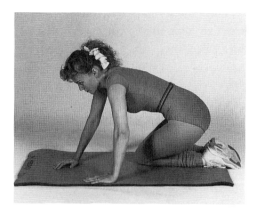

FIGURE 5.10

THIGH STRETCHES
Muscles stretched: quadriceps

Stand on the left leg. Bend the right leg and grasp the ankle (not the foot) with the opposite arm. If you have difficulty grasping with the opposite arm, the same arm can be used if the following alignment is maintained.

Keep the knee pointed downward. Allow a comfortable knee bend and pull gently backward at the ankle. (The right foot should not be forced to the right buttocks.) Maintain good posture and alignment by pulling in the abdomen and keeping the pelvis straight. Avoid arching the back or leaning forward. To keep your balance extend the free arm to the side or overhead, look at something stationary, and keep the abdomen pulled up (Figure 5.11a). You can also place the extended hand against a wall or on a partner's shoulder. This same stretch can be performed lying on your side on the floor (Figure 5.11b).

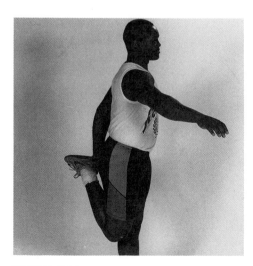

FIGURE 5.11a

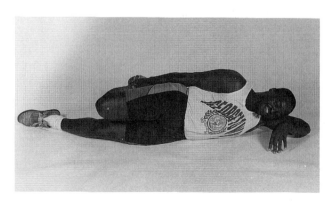

FIGURE 5.11b

BACK OF THE LEG STRETCHES
Muscles stretched: hamstrings

Exercisers have traditionally stretched the muscles at the back of the legs by performing a standing toe touch. Today, sports medicine professionals are concerned that hanging in this position stresses the ligaments that support the back, which could result in lower back pain. When the knees are straight, most of the major muscles in the hip and lower back area cannot function effectively to support the back. Bending the knees helps relieve the pressure on the lower back and allows the muscles to aid the ligaments. But, like the side stretch, hanging in one direction for an extended amount of time places stress on the intervertebral discs. Rather than hang in forward flexion, the toe-touch position, you can use some alternative methods of stretching the hamstrings. Some of these alternatives are:

1. Sit on the floor with the legs extended forward. Bend the left knee and place the left foot flat on the floor. Hold the bent leg and pull yourself gently forward (Figure 5.12). If this is uncomfortable, place the hands behind the buttocks for support and try sitting up straight. This sitting position is good for inflexible people. More flexible people may not feel a stretch in this position.

2. Lying flat on the back, extend the right leg straight out, bend the left leg, and place the left foot flat on the floor. Lift the right leg up until you feel the hamstring stretching. Keep the knee facing the chest; don't turn it out (Figure 5.13a). Use the thigh and hip muscles to pull the right leg toward your head. By contracting the quadriceps muscle, you are allowing the hamstrings to relax and stretch (antagonist stretch technique). The hands should assist only slightly, if at all.

   The lower leg can also be straightened along the floor as long as this does not cause the lower back to strain or lift up off the floor. Use a towel if you have difficulty reaching the leg (Figure 5.13b). Assisted stretching can be achieved by having a trustworthy partner push slowly and steadily against the leg. Partners must listen carefully to each other and push the leg only to a point of mild discomfort.

3. Stand with the right leg bent and the left leg extended forward with the heel resting on the floor or step (bench). With hands on the thigh of the right leg, bend forward at the waist (Figures 5.14a, 5.14b).

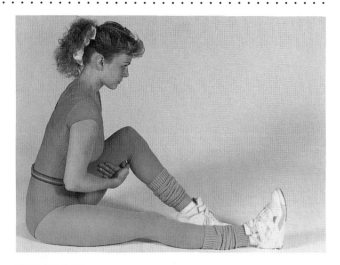

FIGURE 5.12

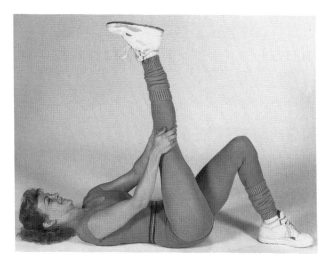

FIGURE 5.13a

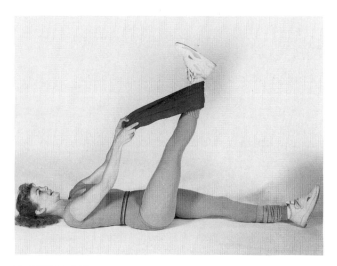

FIGURE 5.13b

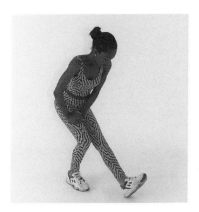

FIGURE 5.14a

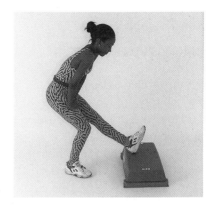

FIGURE 5.14b

INNER THIGH STRETCHES
Side Lunge Position (Legs to the Sides)
Muscles stretched: adductors, gracilis

With your body facing forward assume a lunge position with right knee bent and left leg extended. Both feet should be comfortably aligned with the knees. As in the previous lunge position the bent right knee

should not extend beyond right instep. Hands are placed on the floor in front of body for support (Figure 5.15a). Try to lower hips. When a bench (step) is used, straddle the bench and place hands on top. Less flexible individuals may find this position more comfortable (Figure 5.15b).

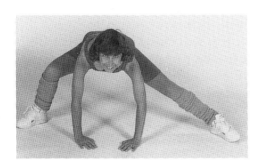

FIGURE 5.15a

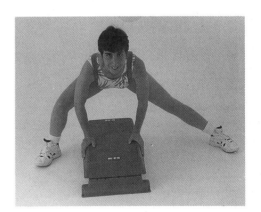

FIGURE 5.15b

Butterfly Position
Muscles stretched: adductors, gracilis

Sit on the floor with the soles of the feet together. Grasp the ankles. (Grasping the toes and pulling may stress the ligaments of the feet.) It is usually most comfortable to grasp the right ankle with the left hand and the left ankle with the right hand. Sit up tall and lean forward until you feel a stretch in the groin area (Figure 5.16). Touching the head to the feet stretches the lower back instead of the groin area.

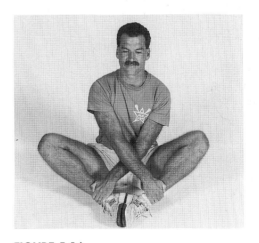

FIGURE 5.16

Modified Straddle Position
Muscles stretched: adductors, gracilis

Sit on the floor with the left leg extended and the right leg bent in front. Stretch forward from the base of the spine (Figure 5.17). Think of putting your nose on the floor as far in front of you as possible.

You can also use this exercise to stretch the back of the legs by turning the hips to face the extended left leg and stretching forward. This is called the modified hurdler's stretch.

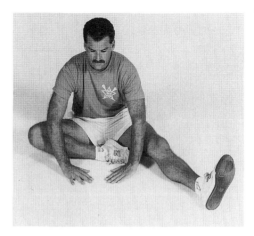

FIGURE 5.17

COMBINATION LEG AND HIP STRETCH
Front Lunge Position
(One Leg Forward, One Back)
Muscles stretched: quadriceps, hamstrings, hip flexors

Pretend you are straddling a straight line. Place the left foot out in front of your body just to the left of the imaginary line. Bend the left knee. Extend the right leg straight back with the right big toe just to the right of the line. Keep the hips absolutely square. Place your hands on the floor (or bench) one on each side of the bent leg to support your weight. Try to lower the hips toward the ground (Figures 5.18a, 5.18b). The bent front knee should stay above or behind the instep. (When the knee is pushed forward and the heel of the front foot lifts, stress is placed on the knee ligaments.) When you want more stretch, move the rear foot back.

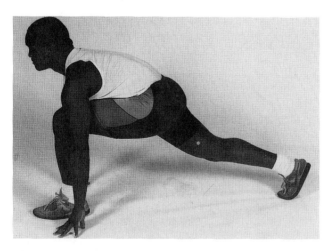

FIGURE 5.18a

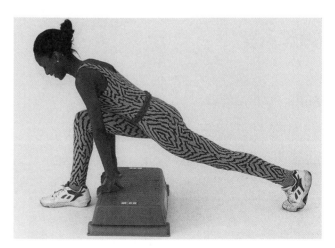

FIGURE 5.18b

HIP STRETCHES
Muscles stretched: hip flexors

1. Place the legs in a front lunge position with the left foot in front. The back toes face straight ahead. The front foot may be turned slightly inward for balance. The back heel is off the ground. Keeping the hips square and the pelvis tucked under, try to lower the hips. Be sure the front foot is far enough out in front to do this comfortably. To avoid ligament stress, the bent front knee should stay directly above or behind the instep. The hands can be placed on the hips or on the front leg (Figure 5.19a). This same stretch can be achieved in a kneeling position (Figure 5.19b). You may want to pad the knees with a towel or mat.

2. You can also stretch the hip flexors while lying on your back. Grasp under the knee and pull one leg to the chest while keeping the other leg straight along the floor (Figure 5.20a). The extended bottom leg results in a greater stretch to the iliopsoas muscle (vs. the quadriceps) than the previous two positions. Both the quadriceps and iliopsoas are hip flexors. Even more iliopsoas stretch can be achieved using a bench (Figure 5.20b).

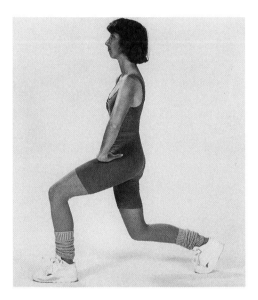

FIGURE 5.19a

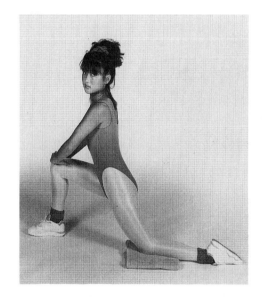

FIGURE 5.19b

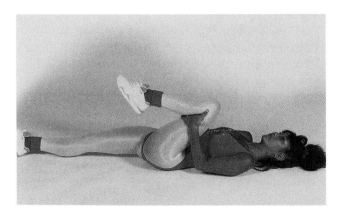

FIGURE 5.20a

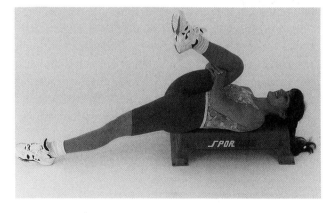

FIGURE 5.20b

BACK/ABDOMINAL STRETCHES
Muscles stretched: erector spinae (flexion), abdominals (extension)

Back flexibility has been neglected in aerobic dance exercise in an overzealous effort to protect the back from pain. Physical therapists and athletic trainers are now encouraging both back flexion and back extension stretching exercises. For lower back flexion lie on the ground and draw both knees toward the shoulders, grasping underneath the knees (Figure 5.21a). For back extension lie face down with the arms bent, resting on the ground with hands up by the ears. Gently press up, supporting your weight on the forearms. Elbows should be under or slightly in front of the shoulders (Figure 5.21b). Hold for 5–10 seconds. If you experience pain, discontinue this exercise and consult a physician.

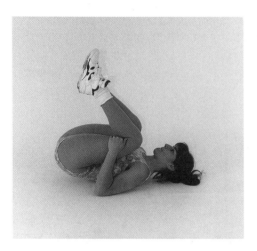

FIGURE 5.21a

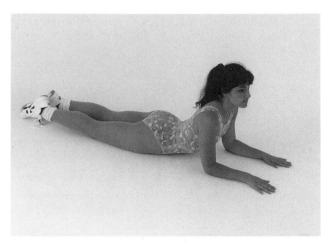

FIGURE 5.21b

CALF STRETCHES
Muscles stretched: gastrocnemius, soleus

Stand in same front lunge position used for hip stretch, but adjust the stance so that back heel touches down. Support or balance yourself by placing hands on the forward knee. Be sure to keep back foot facing directly front and keep the abdomen pulled in. A straight back leg stretches the calf muscle called the gastrocnemius (Figure 5.22a). When you bend the back leg but keep the heel on the ground, you stretch the underneath calf muscle called the soleus (Figure 5.22b).

To perform a calf stretch using a bench (step), stand on top of step. Put weight on right foot bending right knee slightly. Place left foot so that ball of foot is on step but heel is over the edge. Gently press heel down (Figure 5.22c).

You can also stretch calves in a sitting position. Extend one leg forward, keeping knee slightly flexed. Reach forward, grasp toes, and gently pull back. If you can't reach the toes, loop a towel around your foot and pull.

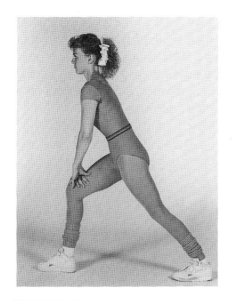

FIGURE 5.22a

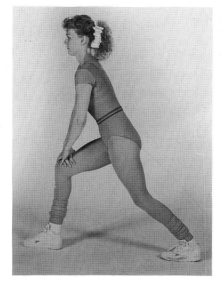

FIGURE 5.22b

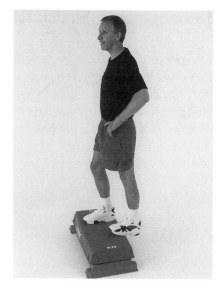

FIGURE 5.22c

COOL-DOWN

Like the warm-up, the cool-down has two sections. The first part, often called the standing cool-down, is done right after the aerobic portion to reduce the body's exertion level gradually from a vigorous activity level. The second portion of the cool-down is the developmental stretch. It will follow either the standing cool-down or a final set of body toning exercises. The purpose of the developmental stretch is to improve flexibility and prevent muscle soreness. The standing cool-down usually lasts 3 to 5 minutes, and the final stretch about 5 to 10 minutes. Time permitting, some instructors will follow the stretch with a few minutes of quiet relaxation.

Standing Cool-Down Technique

During exercise, a large portion of the blood (usually 30 to 50 percent but can be as much as 70 percent) is shunted (circulated out) to the limbs to supply the big working muscles with oxygen. At the end of a workout, it is important to keep moving so the blood is returned to the heart and lungs to be reoxygenated instead of being pooled out in the limbs. If you stop exercising suddenly, you may find yourself feeling light-headed from lack of oxygenated blood in the brain. In fact, fainting is your body's way of getting you level so that the blood doesn't have to be pushed against gravity to get back to the heart, be reoxygenated, and be circulated to the brain. There is no need to feel light-headed or faint in an

aerobics class; simply keep moving and gradually reduce your activity level.

When you move the big muscles of your arms and legs during the standing cool-down, the muscles contract around the veins and help push or massage the blood upward. This aids the **venous pump,** the system of moving blood up through the veins against gravity. Blood is pumped up the **veins** by the pressure created from the heart's contractions. Between heart beats (contractions), blood is held in its newly elevated position by one-way valves inside the veins. Muscle contractions added to the heart's contractions help move the blood more quickly, which in turn helps you recover from exercise more quickly.

When you first start exercising, your aerobic system takes about three minutes to reach a point where it is producing as much energy as you are using. During this time, the anaerobic systems produce energy without the use of oxygen. At the end of exercising, you have to pay back these systems. During the postexercise time, you continue to operate at a high level of oxygen consumption—that's why you continue to breathe hard and sweat after you finish exercising. As everything gets caught up and reset, your breathing and heart rate slow down and you begin to cool off.

The actual movements and technique required for the cool-down are just like the warm-up, only you reverse the process. You'll start with big, active movements and slowly wind down to smaller, easier movements. The key is simply to keep moving; you can even start with a light jog and finish with a walk.

Developmental Stretch Technique

The same stretches and stretch technique used for the opening stretch are used for the closing stretch with one exception: The stretches should be held longer. Although a 10-second hold may improve your flexibility, optimum stretching occurs when you hold for 20 to 60 seconds. The end of class is the best time to do this, since your body temperature is high. Muscles will respond like warm taffy and stretch easily.

. . . .

SUMMARY

Different classes emphasize different things. One class may be composed of very fit individuals who want 30 minutes of aerobics and fewer body toning exercises. Another class may emphasize stretching and toning and do only a 20-minute aerobic workout. In some cases, classes are more or less than an hour long. The short ones will be predominantly aerobic work, while the long ones will have a healthy section of both aerobics and body toning exercises. In all cases, time should be allotted for at least a warm-up, an aerobic workout, a standing cool-down, and a developmental stretch. A well-planned 60-minute class should include the following segments: a 3- to 5-minute core warm-up, a 5-minute sustained stretch (or a 10-minute combined warm-up and stretch), a 20- to 30-minute aerobic workout, a 5-minute standing cool-down, a 10- to 15-minute muscle toning workout, followed by a 5- to 10-minute final (developmental) stretch. If you are late to class, take the time to prepare your body for vigorous exercise. If you must leave early, step out of class with enough time to cool down.

It takes practice to develop good exercise technique. Use the help of instructors, classmates, and mirrors to check your alignment and technique. When you change your technique, it may feel funny or awkward at first, but after a while you will feel better. Be sure to learn both the look and the feel of correctness.

KNOWLEDGE TIPS

1. The warm-up should consist of both a core warm-up and stretching.

2. Use easy movements through a full range of motion during the core warm-up.

3. Hold stretches for a minimum of 10 seconds. Developmental stretching, best done at the end of class, has the greatest effect when stretches are held 20 to 60 seconds.

4. Good technique during an exercise ensures that you will receive the full benefit of the exercise.

5. The standing cool-down is used to bring down your activity level gradually. This activity helps bring blood shunted to the limbs back to the heart.

6. The step (bench) can be used as an effective tool for stretching.

7. The developmental stretch, which occurs at the end of class, develops flexibility and helps prevent soreness.

Rhythmic Aerobics: Variations and Styles

The term *aerobic dance,* which usually conjures up an image of high-impact aerobics, may be too restrictive to describe the great variety of rhythmic activities being done today. Perhaps better described as rhythmic aerobics, the aerobic scene now includes high-impact, low-impact, step, circuit, slide, combat, and aqua (water) aerobics. And this list doesn't even begin to describe all the styles that have developed, everything from funk to yoga aerobics.

The styles of aerobic activity you may encounter vary with the expertise of the instructor. Instructors choreograph low-, high-, or nonimpact routines using their favorite kinds of movements and dance; the results are as varied and as exciting as the instructors themselves.

Victoria Johnson and Christy Lane are both well known for their funky fitness routines done to pop-funk and rap music. Funk is a mixture of ballet, jazz, modern dance, street dancing, maybe some line dancing, and a whole lot of attitude. You can perform funk steps in a style that gets "down and into the floor" or in one that is up, light, and bouncy, called hip hop. Funk can be fast moving and thrilling when you start picking up the moves. (Usually moves are taught at a slower pace and then performed at a fast pace.)

The Salsarobics Company is just one of many that is exploring Latin American dance moves, or salsa moves, on the aerobics floor. Their style combines steps from the merengue, cha-cha, rumba, samba, lambada, and more. Upbeat and wildly popular, country line dancing has also expanded into the aerobic arena. You can get fit doing the Electric Slide or the Achy Breaky.

For those who want to jump less, at least two companies have developed nonimpact aerobic styles. Debby and Carlos Rosas introduced NIA (nonimpact aerobics) as a flowing, undulating, rising and falling form of dance that sustains training zone heart rates with nonimpact changes of feet on the floor. More recently, a company called Yogarobics has applied yoga and tai chi to a new style, which involves moving from a state of quiet or stillness to one of chaotic (vigorous) movements and back to stillness.

Instructors of the martial arts have found a new way to interest people in a great form of exercise—combat aerobics! The actual steps and movements depend a great deal on the instructors, the type of martial arts training they have had, and the experience of the students. Many of the movement patterns involve quick jabbing or kicking movements, so a thorough warm-up is a must. (Some of the martial arts movements traditionally involve deep knee bends. Talk with the instructor concerning modifications if you have or are concerned about developing knee problems.) Combat aerobics may appeal to people looking for self-defense moves. Michael Schwartz kicked off combat aerobics with his Cardio Combat classes. Ken Levy offers Kickboxercise and Thomas Trebotich has developed the BoxAerobic program. It will be interesting to see how popular this activity becomes over the next few years.

To select a class, watch the one you are thinking of joining or take a free trial class. Make sure that the class suits your fitness level and that the instructor is knowledgeable. You may find one style that feels right for you, or with all these possibilities (and more), you may decide to mix it up by using a variety of styles. For example, you might use high-impact or step aerobics as part of your fall sports training, use slide aerobics to prepare for winter sports, use low-impact classes as a change of pace (or when you are pregnant—women only, of course), use aqua aerobics during the hot summer months, and try out salsa-style aerobics before that vacation to Mexico or the Islands.

In this chapter I cannot possibly explain all the styles of aerobics, but I will try to cover the fundamentally different types of rhythmic aerobics: high- and low-impact, step, circuit, aqua, and slide aerobics. If the substantial coverage here (especially of the first three) piques your interest, I encourage you to seek out the wonderful books and training manuals committed to each of these topics. And of course some tremendously talented instructors are standing by to assist you.

THE AEROBICS PORTION OF CLASS

All classes, regardless of type or style have an aerobics portion that conditions your cardiorespiratory system. The training strengthens your heart, reduces the risk of coronary heart disease, reduces your percent body fat, and provides you with a sense of well-being. Some evidence even suggests that aerobic training can lengthen your life, and it definitely can improve the quality. (For a complete discussion of the benefits of aerobic dance exercise, see Chapter 10.)

The aerobic part of class directly follows either the warm-up or any body toning exercises that follow the warm-up. In either case, the first part of the aerobic routine will be moderately paced to bring you up to a training intensity gradually. Instructors often use a low-impact type of aerobics for this first part of the routine. Intensity gradually builds to the most demanding part of the routine, which occurs at the midpoint of the aerobic section. The peak is placed in the middle of the workout because at this stage you are fully warmed up and not yet beginning to fatigue. Following the peak, the level of exertion stays at a training intensity but tapers down as you reach the end of the workout. This aerobic portion of class should be 20 to 30 minutes long (although it may be slightly longer in a low- or nonimpact style of rhythmic aerobics). The aerobic section is followed by the standing cool-down (postcardial section), during which the activity level continues to decrease until you are below your training zone and sufficiently recovered to go on to body toning exercises or a cool-down stretch.

TECHNIQUES THAT APPLY TO ALL RHYTHMIC AEROBICS

1. Maintain good posture. Pull your chin back to prevent jutting your head forward. Pull back gently on your shoulders, pull in your abdomen, keep your hip joint released (relaxed) and vertically aligned, soften your knees, and avoid unnecessarily rounding or arching your back. Pretend you are being pulled up by a string that attaches to the top of your head. Good alignment relieves pressure in your lower back and prevents unnecessary exercise stress.

2. Breathe! Some people have a tendency to hold their breath when they pull in their abdomen. Breathe normally. This means breathing more deeply and quickly as the oxygen demand increases.

3. Keep your feet and knees going in the same direction to prevent rotation soreness, and bend them when landing from a jump. Try to absorb the impact of a jump or step by bending your knees instead of arching your back. (Some people lose their alignment, arching their backs, when they land.)

4. Maintain good back alignment during straight-leg kicks. Aerobicizers tend to exceed the limits of flexibility by kicking too high. To compensate, the lower back will round. Kick only as high as your hamstring flexibility allows. Good kicking alignment is shown in Figure 6.1a, poor alignment in Figure 6.1b.

5. Limit repetition of a movement to a healthy number. This concept is discussed more as it applies to each type of aerobics. For example, in step aerobics you switch lead legs after one minute, and in high-impact aerobics limit yourself to four hops. Repetitions should be limited any time overuse is a concern. If you are recovering from an injury, the number of repetitions may need to be fewer than normal.

6. Control your arm movements. Momentum from flinging an arm can carry the arm beyond its normal range of motion and hurt the joint. Arm movements can and often should move above shoulder level, but the arms should not be held above the shoulders for extended periods of time. The isometric contractions performed by the shoulder muscles will increase blood pressure and may add to unnecessary soreness. Instead arms should frequently move between low, middle, and high positions.

7. Do not wear ankle weights during the aerobic portion of class. Extra weight attached to the ankle increases the risk of impact injury to the lower leg.

8. At this time, physiologists do not recommend the use of wrist weights during the aerobic portion of class. Small wrist and hand-held weights (two pounds) have a very small influence on aerobic work and represent a significant biomechanical danger to the joint if not properly controlled. A fast-moving weight carries more force than a slow-moving weight.

When your movements demonstrate good positioning, alignment, and control, you are said to have "clean lines." It is always fun to watch people with clean lines because they make the movements look crisp and effortless. Strive for this in whichever form of aerobics you select.

HIGH-IMPACT AEROBICS

High-impact aerobics (HIA) classes consist of large-muscle activities such as jogging, jumping, hopping, skipping, knee lifts, dance steps, and calisthenics. Some

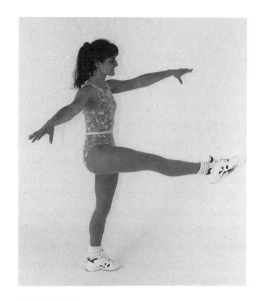

FIGURE 6.1a

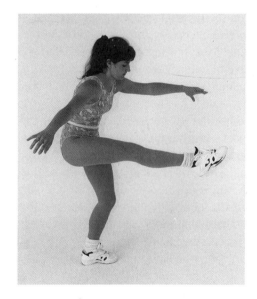

FIGURE 6.1b

routines are highly choreographed; others are improvised. Choreographed routines are not necessarily more dancelike but are simply planned routines that closely follow the music and can be repeated exactly the same way each time. Since they are more planned, well-choreographed routines usually provide a more balanced workout. The advantage of free-style routines is their spontaneity and easy adjustment to class ability.

Planting the foot is probably the most important skill to perfect, since many HIA steps require you to land on the balls of your feet. A dancer counts four different positions between being on the ball of the foot and standing flat. Although you don't need to be able to identify the four positions, you do need to learn how to roll down through all of them as you land from a jump. To land, roll down through the balls of your feet (Figures 6.2a and 6.2b) and bend your knees as you touch down your heels (Figure 6.2c). When you forget to touch your heels down, your calf muscles remain contracted. Constant contraction for 20 to 30 minutes makes for very tight calf muscles. Rolling your feet all the way down will also help prevent shinsplints.

Moderation is the key. Since you are bringing three to five times your body weight down on your foot each time you hop, it is a good idea to limit the number of consecutive repetitions on one foot to four hops. This moderation will help prevent overuse injuries such as **shinsplints** and **tendinitis.** Similarly, overdoing two-footed movements can be hard on the lower legs. Switch off two-footed steps with steps that involve alternate feet. Lateral leg movements, such as jumping jacks, press the knee and ankle in an outward direction. They are good exercises, but you should limit the number you perform in a row, and you should bend your knees as you land. If at any time you feel overuse occurring, modify the routine you are doing. Most instructors will be glad that you took the initiative to individualize your workout.

During a running stride there is a point at which both feet are off the ground. This float time allows the legs to momentarily escape impact stress. Whenever room permits, high-impact choreography should include float time. Even if instructors do all of their steps in place, you can move around a little and pick up the benefits of float time. Big circle formations are wonderful for allowing participants to stride it out. When given the opportunity, run in a normal heel-toe fashion because this movement allows your calves to stretch out.

Often instructors will have the class jog in place while working on arm movements. During this time pay special attention to foot plant and leg position. Relaxing technique—kicking your heels out to the side or letting your knees turn out—is easy. Instead, concentrate on technique—lift your knees directly to the front and roll down through your foot with each step.

LOW-IMPACT AEROBICS

Low-impact aerobics (LIA) is designed to provide an aerobic experience without the risk of injury that may result from the stress of high-impact movements. To accomplish this goal, one foot must touch the floor at all times. Keeping one foot on the ground effectively cuts in half the impact stress. In place of the jumping movements of HIA, LIA substitutes bending movements that lower and then raise the body's center of gravity. Because of the lessening of impact shock, LIA is a good activity for people who are prone to shinsplints, but both the bending and the lateral steps often associated with LIA may irritate a knee joint that is prone to injury.

LIA participants can increase their workout intensity by moving their body's center of gravity upward against gravity. When you jump you move your center of gravity up however many inches you jump. In LIA, you bend your knees, lowering your center of gravity, and then lift it upward by returning to your starting position or perhaps higher by rising up on the balls of your feet. The sinking and rising motions of LIA are one way in which work is created. Large, controlled arm movements moving through a range of motion that includes overhead positions also increase intensity, since work above the heart is more difficult for the body. Extended limbs (long levers) are also more challenging to move than are bent limbs (short levers). For example, swinging the arms out to the

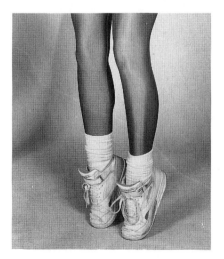

FIGURE 6.2a

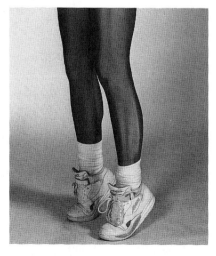

FIGURE 6.2b

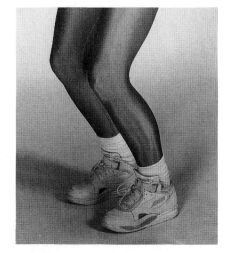

FIGURE 6.2c

side and then overhead is more difficult when the arms are extended than when they are bent at the elbow. Finally, large moving patterns are effective for raising the heart rate. Think of the energy expended in long, striding steps such as those used in power walking. Traveling moves can go side to side, forward and back, on the diagonal, or in a circle. The larger the space you have to work out in, the more you can take advantage of traveling steps.

Technique pointers for LIA include (1) turn your feet and knees out during large (wide) steps to the side—this placement helps maintain hip, knee, and foot alignment; (2) make sure knee flexion does not exceed 90 degrees; and (3) avoid too many steps that cross the foot in front while moving to the side (such as the "grapevine" step), since this type of movement can promote pronation.

The music for LIA is moderately paced (120–140 bpm) to allow sufficient time to execute larger movements. Occasionally instructors use slightly faster music, for which they may increase the speed of dance steps and decrease the size of steps or movements. LIA choreography should follow natural movement patterns and be performed with good muscle control.

One of the advantages to LIA is its emphasis on arm work. Most women lack good upper-body strength, as is evident in the number of women who can perform just one pull-up. LIA and some good upper-body resistance exercises can improve upper-body strength.

Another advantage of LIA is that more people can do it than HIA. LIA is ideal for people who are overweight, since jumping with extra body weight puts excessive strain on joints. It is also good exercise for elderly people who no longer enjoy jumping and for those who experience incontinence with jumping. Large-breasted women and women in a pre- or postnatal condition may also prefer this less bouncy exercise. People who tend to have chronic impact stress injuries as well as people returning to exercise after an injury may prefer LIA. In addition, HIA exercisers may enjoy LIA for a change of pace. It is also a less stressful class for individuals who demonstrate poor biomechanical technique or who have poor structural leg alignment. And it provides a comfortable way for beginners to start, since LIA is easy to adapt to a low-intensity workout. Under a physician's care, people with high blood pressure, heart problems, orthopedic problems, or physical disabilities can enjoy a LIA class although participants with a special medical condition should check with their physicians before beginning a class. LIA may also be a good way for people with diabetes and asthma to start exercising, since they can increase their workout intensity gradually. Once these individuals know how exercise will affect them, they can work up to a high-intensity

LIA or HIA class. Because LIA is so adaptable, it appeals to people of all ages, often bringing together one, two, or even three generations.

STEP AEROBICS

Step aerobics (also called bench) was invented and popularized by Gin Miller in the late 1980s. She then teamed up with Reebok to create the Step Reebok program, which includes guidelines for both teaching and performing step aerobics. Step aerobics consists of patterns of stepping up and down on a bench that is between 4 and 12 inches high. Bench height is adjusted according to the participant's fitness level: lower for beginners and higher for more advanced students. One of the biggest advantages to step training is that people of different fitness levels can perform the same steps to the same tempo side by side—the bench height and arm movements determine the intensity. This has become the most popular form of aerobic dance exercise for men. Some instructors use very clean, almost military-looking movements, while others use more dancelike movements. Stepping patterns start out very simple and build in complexity. Some instructors even use two benches per person and take the steps up and down across both. Although this practice adds a lot of fun variations, it does not increase the aerobic effect, and it requires twice as much equipment and space.

Step aerobics can be performed on the floor (lowest level intensity), on a low step, or on a higher step for a higher intensity (see Figure 6.3).

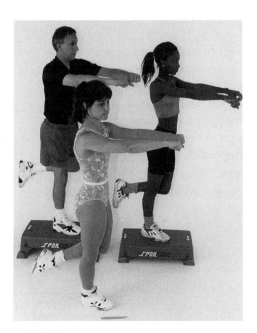

FIGURE 6.3

BASIC STEPS FOR STEP AEROBICS

The leg you step with first is referred to as the *lead leg*. Usually, you begin a new step with the right leg. Since it's best not to lead off with the same leg for more than one minute of stepping, you'll use a *tap change* to change from one lead leg to the other. The tap change is explained and diagrammed below.

In these diagrams, all steps will be presented with an initial right-leg lead. The right foot has been shaded to help you distinguish between right and left legs. When necessary an aerial view of the step has also been included. Most steps are performed in four counts, although positions between counts are also shown for clarification. The positions you should be in on the count are labelled.

Basic Step

Step 1

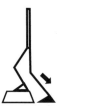

Face step.

Step 2

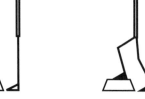

Place right foot on step. (count 1)

Step 3

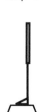

Bring left foot up.

Step 4

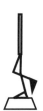

Place left foot next to right foot. (count 2)

Step 5

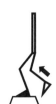

Shift weight to left foot.

Step 6

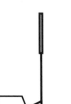

Step down with right foot. (count 3)

Step 7

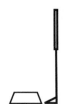

Step down with left foot. (count 4)

Tap Change

The basic step illustrated above was performed with a right-foot lead. To change to a left-foot lead perform the tap change in the alternate Step 7. This tap allows you to lead with the left foot for the next basic step. Tap changes may be used to change the lead leg after one step or after a series of different steps.

Step 7 alternate

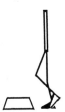

Tap left toe on floor without putting weight on it, then lead with left foot in next step.

V-Step

This step is the same as the basic step, but the feet are positioned further apart on the bench and closer together on the floor. An aerial view helps demonstrate this.

Basic step

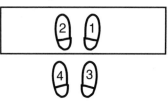
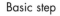

V-step

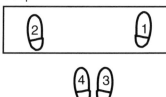

Knee-Ups

The basic step can also be performed with a leg curl, a forward leg kick, or a side leg lift.

Step 1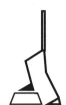

Face step.

Step 2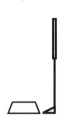

Place right foot on step. (count 1)

Step 3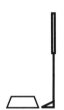

Bring left leg up without touching step.

Step 4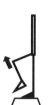

Continue to draw left leg up to knee-up position. (count 2)

Steps 5 and 6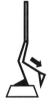

Reverse steps 3 and 4 and place left foot on floor. (count 3)

Step 7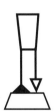

Bring right foot down next to left foot. (count 4)

Tap Up, Tap Down

Step 1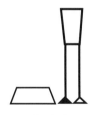

Stand sideways to step.

Step 2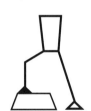

Place right foot on step. (count 1)

Step 3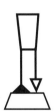

Bring left foot up and tap it on step. (count 2)

Step 4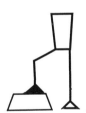

Step down with left foot. (count 3)

Step 5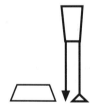

Step down with right foot and tap it on floor. (count 4)

Over the Top

Step 1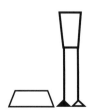

Stand sideways to step.

Step 2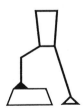

Step up with right foot.

Step 3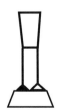

Step up with left foot and shift weight onto it.

Step 4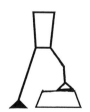

Step down with right foot.

Step 5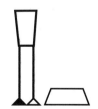

Step down with left foot.

Straddle Down

Step 1	Step 2	Step 3	Step 4	Step 5

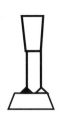 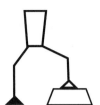 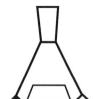 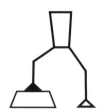

Stand on step facing end.

Step down to right with right foot. (count 1)

Step down to left with left foot, straddling step. (count 2)

Step up with right foot. (count 3)

Step up with left foot. (count 4)

Corner to Corner

Step 1	Step 2	Step 3	Steps 4 and 5

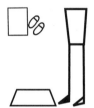 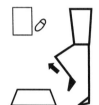 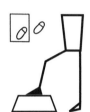 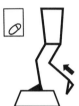

Face left corner of step.

Lift right (inside) leg.

Place right foot diagonally on corner of step. (count 1)

Draw left leg into knee-up position. (count 2)

Step 6	Step 7

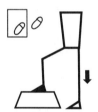 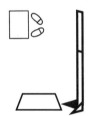

Step down with left foot. (count 3)

Step down with right foot and turn toward right corner of step. (count 4)

Continue the corner-to-corner pattern using the right corner of the step. Count 1 equals place left foot diagonally on corner of step. Count 2 draw right leg into knee-up position. Count 3 step down with right foot. Count 4 step down with left foot and turn toward the left corner of the step.

Toe Tap

Step 1	Step 2	Step 3	Step 4

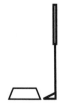 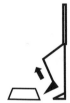 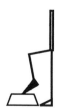 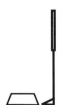

Face step.

Lift one leg.

Tap step with toe. (count 1)

Return to beginning position. (count 2)

Classes begin with an off-the-bench warm-up and then slowly bring up the intensity. The progression pattern most often used is one of learning the step pattern, adding arms, and then adding a direction change. For example, you might begin with a basic pattern of stepping on and off the bench, add arm curls with each step, and then turn the stepping so that you are stepping on the diagonal (corner to corner). Depending on the level of the class, the instructor may stop the arm motion until the new direction is established and then may restart the arm motion or begin a new arm motion. The stepping portion of class is followed by an aerobic cool-down, which finishes with off-the-bench steps and then some strength and flexibility work. The bench is a useful tool for strength and flexibility moves such as the triceps push-ups (p. 70, Fig. 7.25) and hamstring stretch (pp. 38 and 39).

Step training is fun and easy to do. Here are some technique tips to get you started:

1. Place your whole foot on the bench. Be careful the heel of your foot is not overhanging the near edge.

2. Lean from your ankles, not your waist.

3. Step down near to the bench.

4. Roll down through your foot (toe, ball, heel) unless you are doing lunge steps or repeaters, in which case touch only the ball of your foot down.

5. Look where you are stepping by keeping your head up and using your eyes to look down.

6. Wear shoes that have a heel notch to avoid irritation of the Achilles tendon.

7. Before stepping, warm up calf muscles well.

8. Adjust the step height to match your fitness level. Never use a step that bends your knee more than 90 degrees.

9. Adjust workout intensity by increasing or decreasing arm use and extension.

10. Decrease intensity by performing steps off the bench if you become fatigued.

11. Change lead legs after a maximum of one minute.

12. On repeater steps perform a maximum of five repetitions. Here is an example of a repeater step: Step onto the bench with the left foot, draw the right knee up in a knee lift, touch the ball of the right foot to the floor, draw the right knee back up in a knee lift, touch the right ball of the foot to the floor, knee lift again, step down right, step down left. The three knee lifts constitute three repetitions.

13. If you are working at an advanced level and are using power/propulsion moves, perform the moves for approximately one minute (or less) and then alternate with a less stressful step.

14. When performing a kick or a lunge to the back, be careful about placing your arms high overhead, as this movement may lead to back arching.

15. Step quietly. Stamping or stomping on the step will increase impact stress—unless, of course, you are so mentally stressed that the release is well worth the added leg stress!

Caution: This activity is *not* recommended for people with knee joint problems unless a physician prescribes it.

Pages 50–52 provide a visual and written description of the basic movements for step aerobics.

AQUA AEROBICS

Aqua (water) aerobics is a great way to get all the benefits of an aerobic workout with motivating music, a cool environment, and little or no impact stress. And anyone of any age and fitness level can do it. Like step aerobics, this activity can be easily modified so people of different abilities can exercise at the same time. Unlike swimming, in aqua aerobics you do not have to get your hair wet—unless it is very hot out, in which case wetting your hair will help keep you cool.

An aqua aerobics class is very similar to any other aerobics class. Class includes a warm-up (which may be done in the water or on deck), a stretching session, an aerobic portion, an aerobic cool-down, a muscle toning session, and finally flexibility work. Because the water gives you buoyancy, which in turn decreases the impact stress as you push off the bottom of the pool, the aerobics portion of the class can be extended with less risk of injury. Of course, participants must still be careful to avoid joint overuse.

Water is 12 times more resistive than air, so exercisers expend energy by pushing and pulling against this resistive force. For example, it would be 12 times harder to walk through water than through air; hence you will burn more calories walking through water. Aqua aerobic movements are designed to provide balanced muscle workouts. If you pull up with your arm using your biceps, then you will also push back down against the water using your triceps.

All of the principles of exercise you've learned in this book apply to exercise in the water. Many of the regular aerobic exercises can be used in the water. But there are some significant differences, and a few are listed here:

1. Be sure that your music source runs on batteries, not electricity. You can also purchase a Walkman designed for the pool.

2. Heart rates in the pool will be about 10 to 15 percent lower than those on land, largely because your body cools more easily in water, resulting in less work for the circulation system. The more submerged you are, the more this will be true. Water pressure also helps aid venous return, and buoyancy reduces the effects of gravity.

3. Dehydration may occur more easily. Most classes are held outdoors in warm weather or indoors in a heated area. Because you are in water you may not realize how much you are sweating. Drink water from a plastic container (glass is not allowed in pool areas) throughout class. Much of your body's heat is lost through your head, so be careful wearing a swimming cap that traps in heat as it may cause heat stress in warm weather. If you are in a pool that requires a cap (to help keep hair from clogging the pool filter) and you don't mind getting your hair wet, you can wear a Lycra cap and get it wet periodically.

4. Pool attire might seem obvious, but here are a few tips to consider. If you get cold easily, wear tights and a suit or leotard in the pool. Wash out clothing immediately after changing—chlorine is very hard on fabrics. Lycra blends tend to hold up better in pools. Women may prefer one-piece suits with a good built-in bra for support when jumping. Purchase a pair of aqua shoes, which prevent abrasions caused by pushing off the pool bottom, provide cushioning, and supply traction in and out of the pool.

5. Equipment such as webbed gloves and plastic or foam barbells can be used to increase resistance. For deep-water work, you can use flotation belts, jogging vests, kick boards, and other devices to support your body while you are performing running-type exercises. Some devices are contoured better than others to fit comfortably under your arms.

6. You will feel more impact stress when you jump in shallow water than in deep water because you have more buoyancy in deep water.

7. Music tempo is usually between 124 and 136 bpm but with a highly conditioned class may be as high as 150 bpm.

8. When speed is added to a movement, resistance (intensity) increases. When speed is reduced, intensity decreases, but larger ranges of motion with more extended limbs can occur. A variety of movements and movement speeds encourages a good overall workout.

9. Optimum water temperature is between 83 and 86 degrees F. Cool water is good for people with multiple sclerosis, whereas warmer water is good for people with arthritis. Hot water would be good only for a class performing stretching movements.

10. Intensity may be increased or decreased in a number of ways. See the discussion in Chapter 8 on pages 83–84.

Aqua aerobics has become popular and has expanded into a variety of forms. Some classes resemble aerobic dance exercise, some use a weighted step for aqua step aerobics, others have participants run in deep water, and some use circuit- and interval-training principles. As a side note, race horses have been doing deep-water running in harnesses for years. Trainers know that they can train the horses longer and harder without risking stress fractures. So you see, you, your family, and your horse can all perform aqua aerobics together!

CIRCUIT AEROBICS

Circuit training has been around a long time and is now being applied to the new varieties of aerobic training. The idea behind circuit training is that a series of exercise stations are set up in a specific order. The participant progresses from one station to the next, with or without a rest, depending on the type of training desired. The circuit can consist of stations of any type: aerobic, anaerobic, flexibility, muscular strength, or endurance. If the purpose of the circuit is to train the aerobic system, then an all-aerobic circuit is desirable. This way continuous, large-muscle, rhythmic activity occurs for 20 to 60 minutes. Such a circuit might have in it an exercise cycle, a rowing machine, a stair machine, a jump rope, a minitrampoline, a slide board, and a treadmill. Or it might be composed completely of aerobic dance–exercise step patterns. For example, one station might be knee lifts, the next might be four jumping jacks and four kicks, and the next might be a series of steps onto a bench.

A mixed circuit might consist of stations such as push-ups, curl-ups, and leg lifts interspersed between aerobic stations. Although this can be effective training, you must be careful not to drop your head down after vigorous aerobic work, since lowering your head may cause light-headedness, and you should be careful in using weights when fatigued from another station.

It may be smart to take short recovery breaks between stations. When you take rest breaks between stations or between two sets at one station, you are using **interval training.**

Interval training is very good for developing the cardiorespiratory system but not necessarily for developing the aerobic system. For interval training to be effective, exercisers must perform intense work followed by a short rest (anywhere from 10 seconds to one or two minutes). This type of conditioning emphasizes the anaerobic system. To make significant cardiorespiratory gains, the anaerobic work must occur at about 80 to 90 percent of your heart rate reserve. This level is uncomfortable for most people, increases the chance for injury, and does not promise the fat-burning benefits associated with aerobic conditioning. Using interval or circuit training at lower levels will not produce cardiorespiratory training (except for people at a very low fitness level) but can provide good muscle strength and endurance. People interested in circuit training can also increase muscle strength and endurance by using weight-lifting equipment.

SLIDE AEROBICS

Slide aerobics is relatively new and is catching on mostly as a way to stay fit at home, but some clubs and schools have adopted it. Ice skating (speed skating) done at an appropriate target heart rate certainly provides high-quality cardiorespiratory conditioning. The slide provides you a way to perform these skating-type motions without hosing down your living room floor and turning down the thermostat. Two of the greatest features of slide aerobics are that it is a very low- to nonimpact activity and that it can be performed at low to high intensities. The gliding motion, which is easy on the lower legs, is a wonderful lower-body workout and is especially good for toning the inner thighs. Disadvantages to the slide are that feet tend to stick on cheap boards, the activity is somewhat repetitive, and sliding is done individually, not socially, unless you get together with other slideboard owners. Overuse can also occur if you don't

use both side-to-side and forward-and-back movements or if you don't overload gradually. Some instructors like to offer a combination step and slide class. This cross training provides a well-rounded muscle workout.

Slide training, or the lateral movement training system, is not new. According to Reebok, speed skaters in northern Europe and Scandinavia 100 years ago took off barn doors, waxed them, put slats on the ends, and glided back and forth. Today slides are used by Olympic speed skaters for conditioning, physical therapists as a rehabilitative tool, and people like us for fun and fitness.

Slides come in several lengths and a variety of prices. Less expensive slides seem to groove more easily and lose some of their glide. More expensive slides have a better surface that holds up over time. All of them will get surface scratches, but that does not affect performance. Adult boards are 5.5, 6, and 8 feet long. Children's slides are 4 to 4.5 feet long, and some therapeutic boards are as small as 2 feet long. A few boards have adjustable ends allowing you to change the length. Shorter boards result in faster steps, while longer boards emphasize strength and power because you have to push off harder. Tall adults should definitely work on an 8-foot board. Boards also come in different widths: Some are 18 inches, others 24 inches wide. When you are first learning, you will tend to move around (up and down) on the slide, and (especially if you have larger feet) you may prefer the wider board. Try one out to see.

Slideboards also have end bumpers to stop your foot. These bumpers should be angled out so that your foot stops in a biomechanically correct position. Some manufacturers bolt the bumpers on while others fuse them on. Bolted bumpers might separate from the slide with use; the second is more expensive but may last longer and cause less trouble.

To glide, you put specially made booties or socks on over your shoes. Shoes should be designed for lateral movement, so a cross-training shoe, a tennis shoe, or most aerobic shoes will work well. You may purchase extra booties, but make sure you have the right kind of bootie for the slide you own.

To get started sliding, you should read the training manual that comes with the slide or learn from an instructor. Start with the basic step and work up to advanced steps. You can work a variety of muscles by changing direction on the mat. In addition to gliding side to side you can turn and glide forward and backward. You can also add a variety of moves to the end of the glide, such as a knee lift or a toe touch. And, of course, you can add arm movements. Depending on how much you bend your knees and how quickly you move back and forth, slide aerobics can be the equivalent of a brisk walk or a hard run. Following are just a few tips to get you sliding.

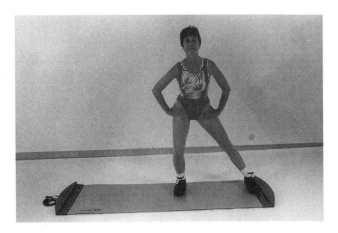

FIGURE 6.4
Pushing off the bumper.

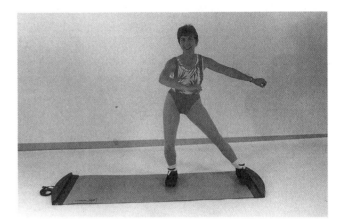

FIGURE 6.7
Pushing off using the arms.

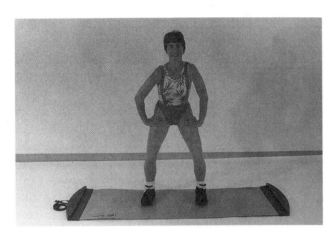

FIGURE 6.5
Gliding across the board.

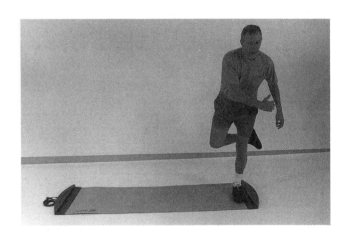

FIGURE 6.8
Pushing off using arms and a leg, similar to a speed skater.

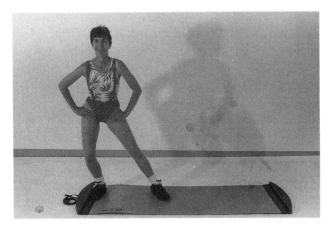

FIGURE 6.6
Stopping on the bumper.

Slideboard provided compliments of Reebok.

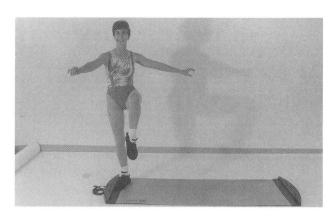

FIGURE 6.9
Ending the glide with a knee lift.

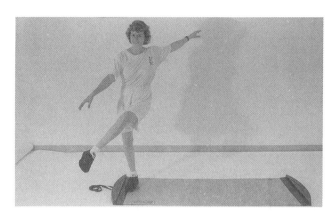

FIGURE 6.10
Ending the glide with a dance "attitude" position.

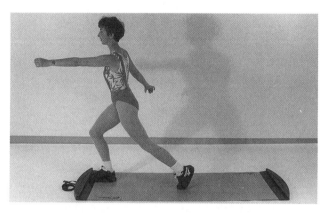

FIGURE 6.11
Pushing off the bumper to glide backward (or finishing a forward glide).

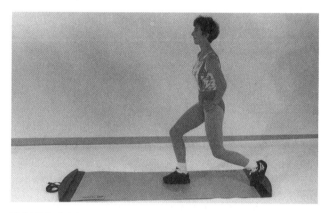

FIGURE 6.12
Ending a backward glide (or pushing off the bumper forward).

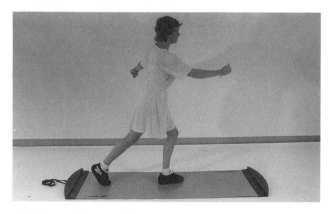

FIGURE 6.13
Cross-country skiing in the middle of the board.

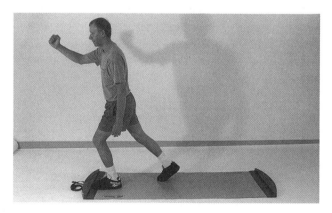

FIGURE 6.14
Cross-country skiing against the bumper.

1. Look at the mat in the beginning and then raise your eyes and look forward or in the direction you are sliding.

2. Keep your knees bent throughout the motion.

3. Lift the outside edge of your foot a little as you approach the bumper—this will help you glide up onto it.

4. Keep your upper body steady, squared to the front, and lean only slightly forward.

Slide aerobics is good for developing the cardiorespiratory system, agility, and balance. You'll need practice to feel balanced, but before you know it you'll be gliding back and forth comfortably.

AEROBICS VIDEOTAPES

Some excellent videotapes are on the market, but some that promote ineffectual or even harmful exercises are also available. Ask your instructor for guidance in selecting one. Also, please be aware that an instructor on tape can't see and correct your body position and technique, whereas live instructors can provide you with this valuable feedback. A combination of live and taped instructors may be the best solution.

SUMMARY

Aerobic dancing has expanded into a family of rhythmic aerobic activities. Some of the newer variations have made it possible for a greater variety of people to get involved. Other variations have resulted in more coeducational classes, and still others have enabled friends of varying fitness levels to exercise together.

KNOWLEDGE TIPS

1. There is more than one right way to achieve aerobic fitness. Select one or more activities that appeal to you.

2. Perform all aerobic movements with good alignment and control.

3. Weights are not recommended for use during the aerobic portion of class.

4. Although all forms of aerobic dance exercise are relatively injury free, some have less impact stress than others.

5. The exercise heart rate during aqua aerobics will be 10 to 15 percent lower than an exercise heart rate out of water.

6. Circuit training involves a series of stations through which the participant moves either with no break or with a short break.

7. Interval training consists of intense bouts of work alternated with short rest periods.

8. You can adjust aerobic intensity by increasing or decreasing arm movements, by raising or lowering the bench height in step aerobics, and by increasing speed or lever length in aqua or high-impact aerobics.

9. New looks in aerobics include slide, funk, combat, yoga, salsa, country, and step aerobics (both in and out of water).

CHAPTER 7

Body Toning Exercises

Body toning exercises are designed to shape, firm, and strengthen the muscles. These exercises are also called strength and endurance exercises, resistance exercises, and floor exercises. Since most people want muscle toning, which is primarily anaerobic, as well as aerobic conditioning, usually 10 to 20 minutes of an hour-long exercise class are devoted to developing strength and endurance. If, however, a class meets for less than an hour the major emphasis should be on aerobic training. Few people die from flabby legs, but it is quite common to die from heart failure. Some people like to supplement their aerobic workouts with one- to two-hour classes designed just for muscle toning. These classes may be offered under different names, such as body sculpting, body building, and body shaping.

Body toning exercises may be performed prior to the aerobic section of class or following the aerobic (standing) cool-down. Professionals are still debating which placement is preferable. Some instructors like to do body toning exercises first, while the class is fresh, and finish on the run. Others like to get the class going with the aerobic portion and finish with the body toning exercises. Still others will incorporate some strength and endurance work both before and after the aerobics segment. Until research demonstrates that one order results in better training than the other, whatever feels good to you is fine.

Body toning exercises can improve both strength and muscular endurance, two of the health-related components of fitness. To understand the relationship between strength and endurance, picture a continuum with one at each end. Exercising with heavy resistance (weight) exhausts muscles in just a few repetitions and builds strength. Exercises of light to moderate resistance performed with many repetitions build muscular endurance.

STRENGTH ◄─────► ENDURANCE

Heavy Resistance | Light-Moderate
Few Repetitions | Resistance
  | Many Repetitions

Because there is no definitive point along the continuum where strength ends and endurance begins, the target zones for these two fitness components overlap. These target zones, like the others presented in this book, are composed of the three FIT variables: frequency, intensity, and time.

FREQUENCY

Individuals wishing to build muscular strength and endurance should do resistance training (body toning, weight lifting) at least twice and if possible three times a week on alternate days. You should not work the same muscle tissue twice in less than 48 hours because the tissue needs time to rest and rebuild. If you work out too frequently, your muscles will weaken over time. Serious weight lifters either work out every other day or exercise one set of muscles one day and a different set the next. The latter type of training is called working split sets.

INTENSITY

Intensity is determined by the amount of resistance involved in the exercise. The more resistance, the greater the force you will have to exert. As depicted on the continuum, muscle endurance activities work with lower levels of resistance than strength exercises. Intensity is measured as a percentage of the maximum weight (resistance) you can lift, push, or pull one time. This weight is often referred to as the **repetition maximum**, or 1 RM. In general, strength gains occur when you work between 50 and 100 percent of 1 RM. Endurance increases when you work between about 20 and 70 percent of 1 RM. These guidelines are easiest to put into use when working with measured weights and weight-lifting equipment. A good rule of thumb is to use an amount of weight or resistance that makes doing 8 to 12 repetitions difficult by the end of the set; this number of repetitions places you in the middle of the strength-endurance continuum. For example, if you can do 8 push-ups on your knees easily but numbers 9, 10, 11, and 12 become progressively more difficult, then you are within the target zone for intensity. When you can perform 12 push-ups

with relative ease, it's time to increase intensity.

You can increase resistance by using more difficult body positions, weights, exercise bands, water, or weight-lifting equipment. Chapter 8 discusses how to add resistance with exercise bands, water, and weights. The following are a few examples of how you can use body position to increase resistance. The easiest push-up to do is one performed against a wall. Place your hands on the wall and put your feet about two feet away from the wall. Bend your arms. You can progressively increase resistance by doing a push-up (1) on your hands and knees, (2) on your hands and toes, (3) on your hands and toes with your hands either very close together or more than shoulder width apart, (4) on your hands and toes but with your toes up on a bleacher or step. You can make side leg lifts more difficult by going from raising a bent leg to raising a straight leg. Curl-ups are easiest with the arms down at the sides of the body, harder with the arms crossed over the chest, and most difficult with the hands up by the head. When an exercise is being performed in class, you should modify the intensity to suit your personal needs.

TIME

Time or duration is expressed in terms of repetitions and sets of repetitions. Experts disagree on the exact numbers of repetitions and sets that build strength or endurance, but in general, one to five sets of 3 to 8 repetitions builds strength and one to five sets of 8 to 25 repetitions builds endurance. For health-related fitness, people often work in the middle of the continuum, performing one to three sets of 8 to 12 repetitions. The ACSM recommends completing a minimum of one set of 8 to 12 repetitions (to near fatigue) of between 8 and 10 exercises that use the major muscle groups. As stated earlier, you should perform these exercises a minimum of two days a week. If you have the time, progressively overload by adding resistance or a second and then third set to your workout. You may also wish to add more exercises to your routine.

You may want to emphasize muscle endurance by performing even more repetitions. The question is, how many repetitions are enough? For example, it is impressive to be able to do 100 push-ups in a row, but does that make you healthier than when you could do 20? To answer this question you need to consider the amount of strength you need for your daily activities, the psychological benefits of being able to perform a certain number, the wear and tear on your body, and the amount of time you have available for training. It is usually more effective to increase resistance and do fewer repetitions than to do a really large number. For good health, attain the amount of strength and muscular endurance you need to perform routine and leisure activities effectively and to function in emergency situations.

Aerobic dance exercise tends to emphasize endurance (toning) over strength (ability to move more weight in one attempt). Exercises are also often performed in multiples of eight in an effort to match music written in 4/4 time. You can personalize your workout intensity and duration by deciding how many repetitions and sets you wish to do and by adding resistance by changing body position or by adding weights and bands.

ISOMETRIC AND ISOTONIC CONTRACTIONS

Isometric contractions occur when the muscle is contracted and the muscle length is held constant. You perform an isometric contraction by holding a weight in one position for a certain amount of time or by exerting a force against an immovable object. The weight being held may be the weight of one of your limbs, your limb plus a weight, or all or part of your body weight. For example, you might hold yourself in a curl-up position for 10 seconds, or you might exert force by pressing one hand against the other. To develop strength using isometric contractions, exert near-maximal force or hold heavier weights for a short duration. To develop endurance hold lighter weights or exert less force for longer durations. Isometric contractions can be very useful for strengthening a muscle in one position, which is particularly helpful in rehabilitation and postural exercises. One important word of caution—isometric contractions result in a rapid rise in blood pressure and are not recommended for people with high blood pressure. Perhaps you've heard of people having heart attacks while trying to push a car out of a snow bank. These people are exerting maximal effort against an immovable object (an isometric exercise), taxing an already stressed cardiovascular system.

Usually, however, you'll want to develop strength and endurance of your muscles through their full range of motion. To do this, perform exercises that use isotonic contractions, also known as dynamic contractions. All of the strength and endurance exercises presented in this chapter are isotonic in nature. They all require that you move through a safe and full range of motion.

TECHNIQUE FOR BODY TONING EXERCISES

While performing these exercises it is very easy to involve more muscles than the ones you are trying to exercise. Isolate the muscle or muscle group you plan to work, use a few others to stabilize your position, and relax the rest.

Perform all strength- and endurance-building exercises at a moderate pace so that momentum will not help do the work. Fast movements strengthen muscles only in the positions where a change of direction occurs. For example, when the arm is quickly raised and lowered, strength is acquired where the arm reverses from an upward movement to a downward one and vice versa. Momentum does most of the work between the turnaround points.

Do not confuse body toning with spot reduction. The idea that a toning exercise will remove fat from a specific body part is false. Only aerobic exercise burns fat. Toning and strengthening exercises work the muscle so that when the fat does burn off, beautifully toned muscles will appear!

The list of exercises presented in this chapter is not all-inclusive. The selected exercises are those commonly performed in aerobic dance–exercise classes. Many of the exercises require that you work first one side of your body and then the other. To save space, the exercise descriptions describe the action for only one side (the side shown in the picture), but you should always work both sides equally.

The names of the muscles being exercised are labeled under each exercise heading. The appendix contains a tear-out diagram of the muscles of the body. You may wish to tear out this diagram and place it alongside the page you are reading so that you can quickly identify the muscles and muscle actions being described.

Although the body toning exercises in an aerobics class predominantly emphasize endurance, strength gains may also occur. These exercises will help you look and feel good. You will be able to do more activities with less fatigue, and the added muscle control will help prevent injuries. If you would like to improve your strength and endurance even more, add weight lifting to your exercise program.

Legs

Two basic positions used in leg exercises require special comment. When working on all fours you can be on your hands and knees (Figure 7.1) or on your forearms and knees (Figure 7.2). In most cases, the latter is recommended because it allows you to lift your leg higher without causing your back to arch. If you are more comfortable in the first position, lift the leg only until it is parallel with the floor.

When you are performing exercises lying on your side, your arm and trunk can be flat along the floor (Figure 7.3) or you can be resting on your forearm (Figure 7.4). Both are fine. If you use the latter, resist the temptation to slouch into the shoulder. Stay pulled up. Lying flat has the advantage of eliminating spinal curvature during the exercise.

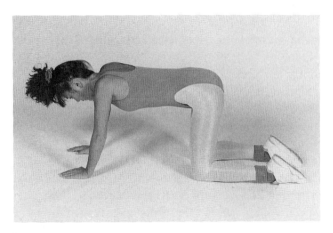

FIGURE 7.1

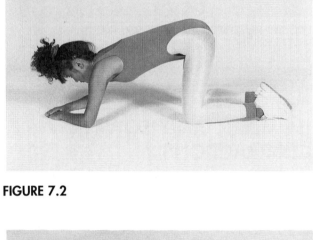

FIGURE 7.2

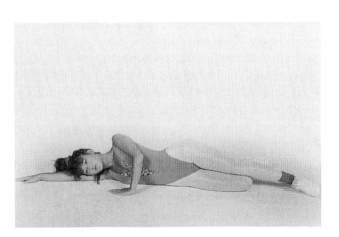

FIGURE 7.3

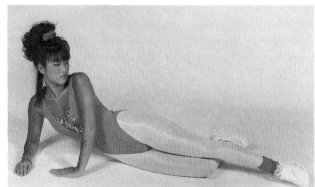

FIGURE 7.4

OUTER THIGH

Muscles worked: abductors

Position 1

Lie on the right side with the left hip directly above the right hip. Keep the upper body flat along the ground or support raised shoulders with the right forearm flat on the floor. The bottom leg may be bent for balance.

Action Lift the top leg straight up and then lower it down (Figure 7.5). Keep the knee facing directly toward the front. (If the knee rotates to the ceiling, the muscles on the front of the leg, instead of the outer thigh muscles, do the work.)

Variations

1. Alternately point and flex the toe.
2. Raise the leg only halfway up and then lower it down (smaller range of motion).
3. Raise the leg all the way up and then lower it only halfway down.

4. Touch the left toe down in front of the right leg (Figure 7.6a). Then rotate and move the left leg so that the left heel touches down behind the right leg (Figure 7.6b). (This will exercise the rotator muscles.)

Position 2

Lie on the right side with the upper body positioned as described in position 1. Bend both knees 90 degrees and flex slightly at the hips for comfort. Adjust the bottom leg for balance.

Action   Raise the top leg and then lower it. Keep the knee facing forward and the lower leg parallel to the ground. (If the knee points toward the ceiling, the muscles on the front of the thigh will work instead of the outer thigh muscles.) I like to call this exercise "accordions" (Figure 7.7). The bending of the knees requires you to lift less weight than when you keep your legs straight.

Position 3

Support your body on all fours. Keep your weight centered. Elbows should be straight but not locked. The head should be in line with the back. Turn the body sideways to the instructor so that the head can be turned (rather than lifted) to view the instructor. Place

hands shoulder width apart with the fingers facing forward. Pull in the abdomen.

Action   Keeping your weight centered and leg bent, lift the left leg to the side and then lower it (Figure 7.8). Lift until you feel resistance. Do not lift the working hip. If a yardstick was placed on your back, the yardstick would remain parallel to the floor throughout the exercise. Another test to see if your weight is centered is to raise the right arm when the left leg is working. (If the hip is allowed to rise, some of the back muscles are doing the work.) This exercise is often referred to as "hydrants."

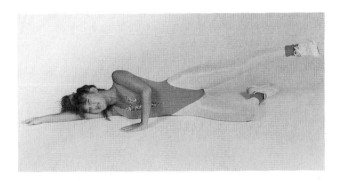

FIGURE 7.5

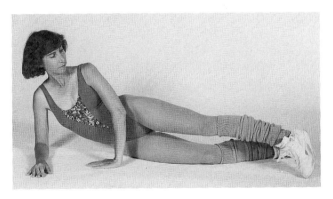

FIGURE 7.6a

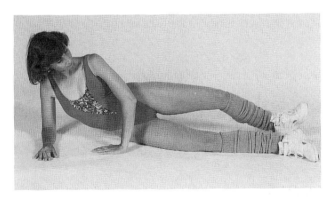

FIGURE 7.6b

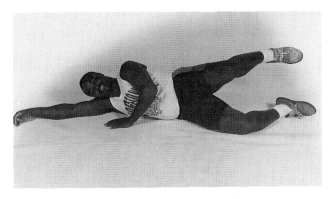

FIGURE 7.7

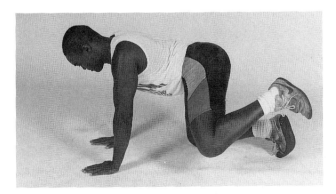

FIGURE 7.8

INNER THIGH
Muscles worked: adductors

Position 1

Lie on the right side. Bend the left leg and allow the knee and lower leg to rest on the floor in front of the body (Figure 7.9a). Keep the left hip directly above the right hip.

A similar position can be used where the left leg is bent, the left foot is in front of the right leg, and the left knee points to the ceiling (Figure 7.9b). Be sure to keep the hips vertical; they have a tendency to roll back in this position.

Action With the inner thigh facing the ceiling, raise and lower the right leg.

Variations

1. Lift the right leg up and slightly back.
2. Flex and point the toe of the right leg when it is lifted off the ground.
3. Circle the right leg forward and then back.
4. Hold the right leg off the ground while bending and straightening the knee (Figure 7.10).

Position 2

Lie on the back. Extend the legs straight up in the air. Straddle the legs and place hands or forearms on the inside of the thighs. (Lack of flexibility may make this uncomfortable for some as it requires the hip flexors and abdominal muscles to hold the legs vertical.)

Action Bring the legs together while resisting with the hands (Figure 7.11), then relax. Start with easy resistance and build up. This exercise can also be done with a partner providing resistance.

Position 3

For people at an advanced fitness level only—may cause lower back strain. Sit up tall with legs extended forward along the floor. Place hands on the floor behind the buttocks. Bend the nonworking leg so that the knee is close to the buttocks. Take the working leg to the side and rotate at the hip so that the inner thigh is facing the ceiling.

Action Raise the leg and then lower it (Figure 7.12).

Variation Raise the leg and then lower it as you move it to the front and then back out to the side.

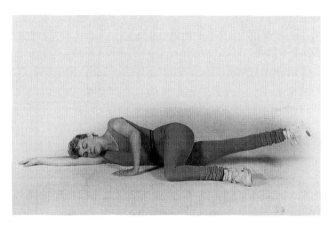

FIGURE 7.9a

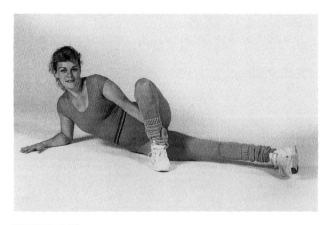

FIGURE 7.9b

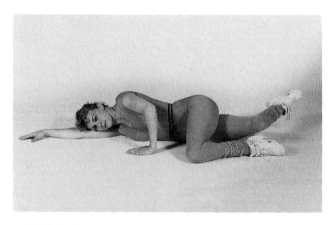

FIGURE 7.10

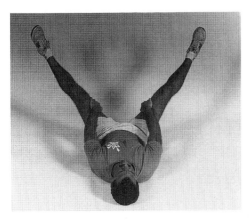

FIGURE 7.11

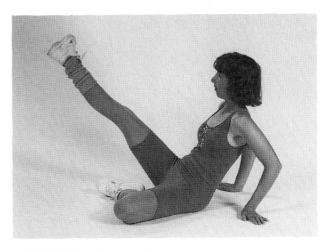

FIGURE 7.12   Advanced.

THIGH

Muscles worked: quadriceps, iliopsoas

Position 1

Assume the crab position (on all fours with the abdomen toward the ceiling). Extend the working leg forward. If the arms get tired, the buttocks can be lowered to the floor.

Action   Lift the leg straight up and then lower it (Figure 7.13).

Variation   Bend the leg in, extend out, lift up, and lower.

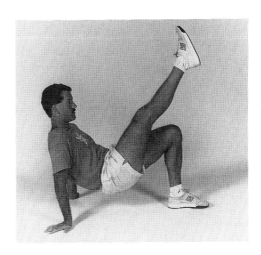

FIGURE 7.13

BACK OF THE LEG

Muscles worked: hamstrings, gluteals

Position 1

Assume the all-fours position (on hands and knees). Lower the shoulders by taking the weight off the hands and onto the forearms. Extend the working leg out to the back. Flex the foot with the heel facing directly up to the ceiling, toes touching the ground (Figure 7.14a).

Action 1   Keeping a straight leg, lift the working leg until it is aligned with the back (Figure 7.14b). Lower and touch the toes to the ground.

Action 2   Lift the working leg until it is aligned with the back (Figure 7.14b). Maintain the knee position, flex the leg, and bring the heel toward the buttocks (Figure 7.15). Then straighten the leg.

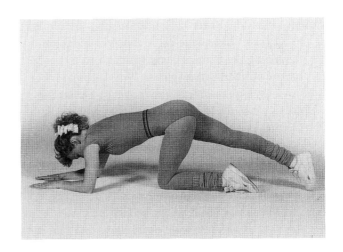

FIGURE 7.14a

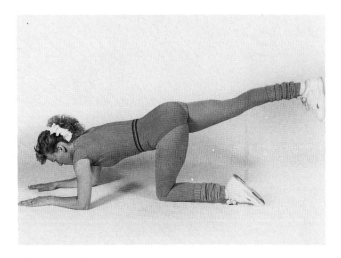

FIGURE 7.14b

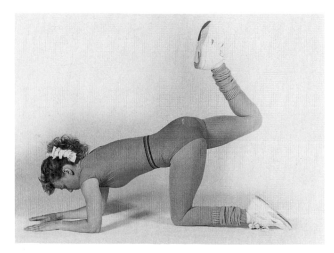

FIGURE 7.15

BUTTOCKS
Muscles worked: gluteals

Position 1

Assume an all-fours position. Lift the working leg up off the floor. Flex this leg 90 degrees. Keep the hips flat. Flex the foot (Figure 7.16a).

Action Keeping the hips flat, lift the leg upward. It probably won't lift very high if you are in a correct position (Figure 7.16b). Lower the leg.

Position 2

Lie on the back with knees bent and feet on the floor about shoulder width apart.

Action Press the lower back into the floor by tilting the pelvis. Continue to roll the pelvis under while tightening the buttocks, and lift the hips a few inches off the floor (Figure 7.17a). Lifting higher involves leg muscles; lifting too high arches the back. When the buttocks are kept tight throughout the movement, it is difficult to lift too high. Roll down and release the pelvic tilt.

Variations

1. Vary the distance between the feet. (Some people feel knee discomfort when the feet are close together. If you feel knee discomfort, don't do this variation.)

2. Start with the knees and feet apart. Draw the knees together during the hip lift. Relax knees as the hips are lowered. You can also hold the hips stable in the lifted position and move the knees in and out. (Again, if you feel knee discomfort, discontinue the exercise.)

3. Cross one leg over the other knee and lift as before (Figure 7.17b) or extend one leg upward and lift as before (Figure 7.17c). When one leg is off the floor, this becomes an advanced exercise, since it is more difficult to roll the pelvis correctly in this position.

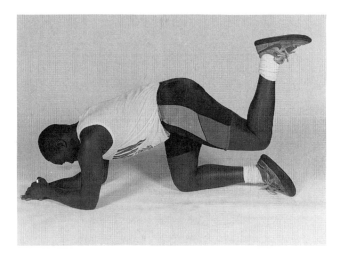

FIGURE 7.16a

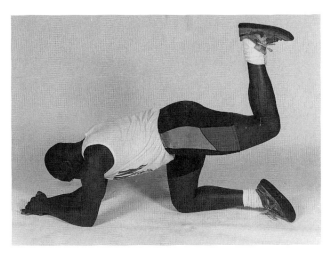

FIGURE 7.16b

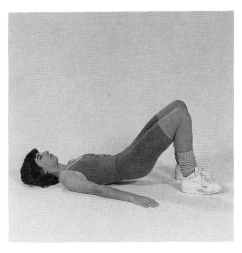

FIGURE 7.17a

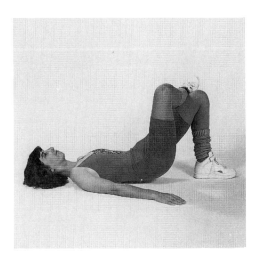

FIGURE 7.17b
Advanced.

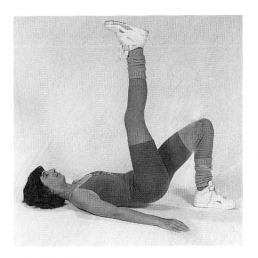

FIGURE 7.17c
Advanced.

COMBINATION EXERCISES

Muscles worked: gluteals, hamstrings, quadriceps

Position 1

Take a large step forward into a lunge position. Keep the knee on the front leg behind the instep of the front foot. Keep hips square.

Action   Lower the hips until the front thigh is parallel to the floor. Take another large step forward to a lunge on the other side and repeat (Figure 7.18).

Position 2

Assume the squat position—feet slightly wider than shoulder width apart, heels down, knees bent, trunk on a forward angle.

Action   Bend the knees to about 90 degrees. Be sure to retain muscular control throughout the movement (Figure 7.19). You should sit backward (as though you are sitting on a chair) and keep the head and eyes forward and slightly raised. Straighten legs and relax.

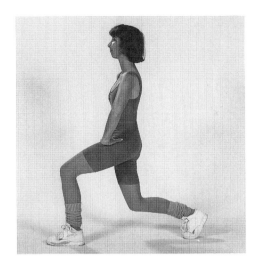

FIGURE 7.18

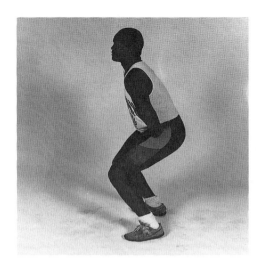

FIGURE 7.19

Arms and Shoulders

You can perform these exercises while standing or sitting. If you stand, the knees should be slightly bent and the pelvis straight or tucked under.

SHOULDERS
Muscles worked: deltoids

Position

Arms extended to the side, elbows straight but not locked.

Action Move the arms in small or large circles first clockwise and then counterclockwise (Figure 7.20).

Variations

1. While circling the arms, move them to the front, overhead, down, and to the side again.

2. With the arms to the side move the arms forward and back with the palms facing forward, then palms back, palms up, and, finally, palms down.

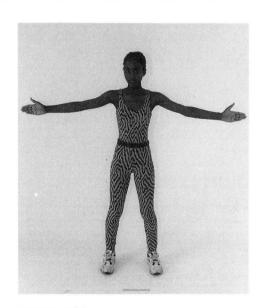

FIGURE 7.20

FOREARMS
Muscles worked: forearm flexors, extensors

Position
Arms are straight and may be down, to the sides, in front, or overhead. Hands may be in a fist or open.

Action   Both wrists can flex, drawing the palm toward the forearm. Both wrists can extend, pulling the back of the hand toward the back of the forearm, or one wrist can flex while one extends (Figure 7.21).

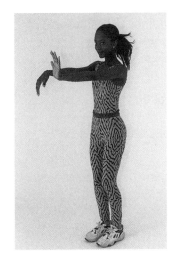

FIGURE 7.21

FRONT OF THE UPPER ARM
Muscles worked: biceps

Position
Arms are relaxed at the sides of the body. Palms should face forward. Hands may be in fists or open.

Action   Flex the arms (Figure 7.22). (Pull the palms or fists toward the shoulders.) Relax and extend the arms.

Variations

1. Hold the arms straight in front of the body parallel to the floor. Flex, relax, and extend.

2. Hold the arms straight out to the sides parallel to the floor, palms forward. Flex, relax, and extend.

3. Hold the arms straight out to the sides parallel to the floor, palms up. Flex, relax, and extend.

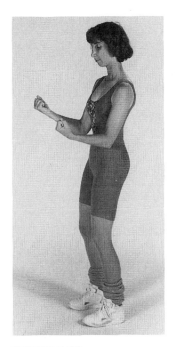

FIGURE 7.22

BACK OF THE UPPER ARM
Muscles worked: triceps

Position 1
Stand with knees slightly bent. Lean the trunk forward slightly. Arms are bent with the elbows drawn up and back. Palms face back (Figure 7.23).

Action   Extend the arms (straighten). Relax, allowing arms to return to the starting position (flexed).

Variation   Rotate the palms 270 degrees to the outside after extending the arm. Rotate the palms back in before lowering the arms.

Position 2

Stand with knees slightly bent. Extend arms straight up overhead. Clasp the hands with the palms facing each other. Leaving the elbows right by the ears, flex the arms, allowing the clasped hands to fall behind the head (Figure 7.24).

Action Extend the arms until they are straight overhead. Relax and return to the flexed position. This exercise is sometimes called the French curl.

Position 3

Assume the crab position, on all fours with the abdomen to the ceiling. You may place the hands on the floor or on a step. (For weak arms place the hands and buttocks on the floor.)

Action Bend the arms to a 90-degree angle (Figure 7.25). Extend arms and return to starting position.

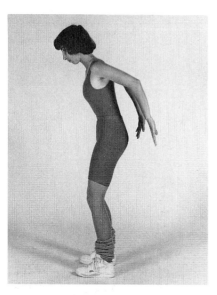

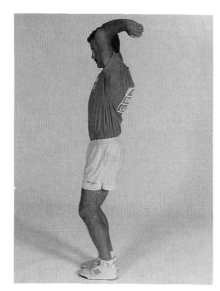

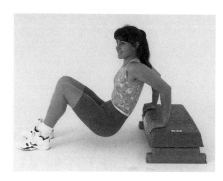

FIGURE 7.25

FIGURE 7.23

FIGURE 7.24

CHEST

Muscles worked: pectoralis major

Position

Stand with the knees slightly bent. Hold the arms out to the side with the upper arms parallel to the floor and the lower arms vertical (Figure 7.26).

Action Bring the arms forward until the forearms touch. Return the arms to the side.

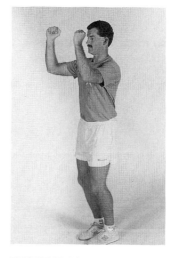

FIGURE 7.26

COMBINATION EXERCISE
Muscles worked: pectoralis major, triceps

Position

Assume the push-up position with hands on the floor, a little more than shoulder width apart. Legs are extended straight to the back with the weight resting on the toes for advanced people (Figure 7.27a). Beginners can rest their weight on their knees (Figure 7.27b). In both cases, the body should be straight with just a slight lift of the gluteals (buttocks).

Action Bend elbows to approximately 90 degrees. Then straighten elbows and return to starting position.

Variations

1. Place the hands farther than shoulder width apart.

2. Place the hands very close together.

3. Place the hands (easier) or feet (harder) on a step (Figure 7.28).

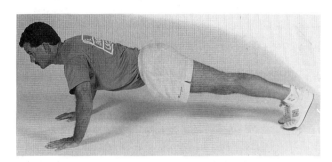

FIGURE 7.27a

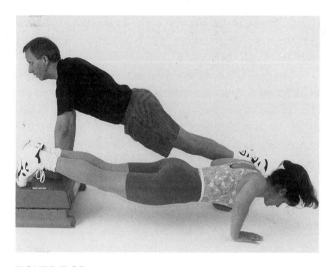

FIGURE 7.28

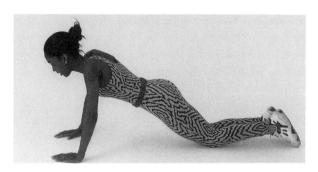

FIGURE 7.27b

Abdominals

A general understanding of the abdominal muscles and their function will help you select specific exercises for your program. The rectus abdominis is a long muscle that attaches to the pubic bone at one end and the ribs at the other. The whole muscle will contract during any abdominal exercise, but some exercises tend to emphasize the upper two-thirds while others emphasize the lower third. The oblique muscles run from the ribs to the pelvic girdle on an angle. When they contract, they twist (or rotate) the trunk with respect to the pelvic girdle. The transversalis is the deepest of the abdominal muscles. It lies underneath both the rectus abdominis and the obliques. Its primary function is postural; practicing good posture by keeping your abdomen lifted and pulled in is the best

way to keep this muscle toned. This muscle is often referred to as the transverse abdominal muscle because the fibers run across the body.

For many years, people have done sit-ups to develop abdominal strength. Sit-ups used to be performed with a relatively straight back and with the hands behind the head. Today, curl-ups are the exercise of choice because they are much easier on the lower back and just as effective as sit-ups. In a curl-up, your head and shoulders follow a natural curl as you lift. (For a while, people were taught to lift the chin straight up; this is incorrect.) You roll up until your shoulder blades come off the floor. If you sit all the way up, your abdominals are resting for the last one-half to one-third of the exercise because the pull of gravity lessens in this range. Your hip flexor muscles also come into action in this range, taking work away from the abdominals.

Arm placement can make curl-ups progressively more difficult. With the arms at the sides of the body, the abdominal muscles are lifting only the weight of the trunk and head. When the arms are placed across the chest, the abdominals must lift the weight of the arms, trunk, and head. When the arms are moved up toward the head, they represent even more weight. Figure 7.29 demonstrates these three positions. An incline board (or bench) can be used for an assisted curl-up (Figure 7.30).

Placing the hands behind the head can be stressful to the neck, and for this reason, many exercise leaders do not use this position. Too often individuals use their arms to pull their body forward, which presses the chin to the chest and stresses the neck. In properly executed curl-ups, the arms remain passive and the abdominal muscles do all the pulling.

The position with the arms near or behind the head is included for two reasons. First, some individuals can clearly maintain good technique and handle the weight of the arms in this position. Second, a few individuals experience neck fatigue prior to abdominal fatigue and like to rest their head in their arms to relieve the neck muscles. However, the vast majority of individuals will achieve the best results by placing their arms alongside their body or across their chest. Weights can also be held against the chest to make curl-ups more difficult.

To concentrate on the oblique muscles you have to twist before lifting the torso. (A common error is to lift and then twist.) One way to ensure good twisting action, when the hands are behind the head, is to leave one elbow flat on the floor while the other lifts across the body.

Strengthening the lower third of the abdomen and not straining the back is a challenge. Eighty percent of all people have back pain sometime during their lives—pain that is often caused by a lack of abdominal strength and leg flexibility. Some exercises seem as though they would increase abdominal strength but in fact may cause lower back pain.

Double leg lifts are one such culprit. A double leg lift requires the abdominal muscles to lift about one-half the body's weight. If the abdominal muscles are too weak to lift both legs, the hip flexors come to the rescue, particularly the iliopsoas. The problem is that the iliopsoas attaches to the spine in the lower back area. When it contracts, it pulls against the lower spine. When the iliopsoas is handling a lot of weight such as in a double leg lift, it pulls the lower back up off the floor, often resulting in lower back pain. Plus, leg lifts that strengthen the hip flexors (iliopsoas and others) and hurt the back fail to do the one thing you set out to do—strengthen the abdomen. Only individuals who possess very strong abdominals and who can keep the lower back on the floor should lift both legs.

Many exercises fall into the "double leg lift" category: straddling the legs six inches off the floor, sitting and pushing both legs out, scissoring at a low angle, and others. Exercises that are better for the majority of the population are single leg lifts, bicycling the legs, or reverse curls. Strengthening the abdominals will help support the spine and decrease susceptibility to back pain. Each of these exercises plus curl-up variations are described here in more detail.

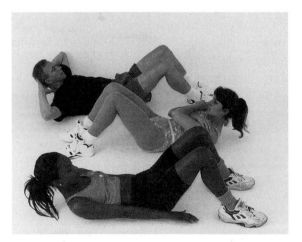

FIGURE 7.29

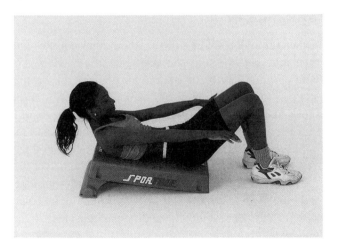

FIGURE 7.30

UPPER ABDOMEN
Muscle worked: rectus abdominis

Position

Assume the curl-up position—lie flat on the back with knees bent, feet flat on the floor and shoulder width apart. Hands may be at the sides, across the chest, or by the head.

Action   Lift the upper body up off the floor while pressing the lower back into the floor. Be sure to lift up and "curl" naturally with the body and neck (Figure 7.29). Roll back down to the floor. Beginners can relax between curl-ups; more advanced participants can curl down until their shoulder blades touch and curl up again.

Variations

1. Lift feet off the floor, ankles crossed or uncrossed, knees bent. Curl up (Figure 7.31). Roll back down to floor.

2. Bend the left leg and place the left foot on the floor. Place the right ankle on the left knee. Perform curl-ups (Figure 7.32). Curl down to floor.

3. Reach for the toes with the legs extended straight up in the air (Figure 7.33). Reach with one hand and place the other behind the head if you experience neck fatigue. The legs can also be bent during the relaxation phase and extended during the reaching phase. Curl down to floor.

4. Bench-assisted curl-up. The angle of the bench helps beginners perform a curl-up (Figure 7.30). Lie down with your back and buttocks on the angled bench and your feet on the floor. (Tall people may have difficulty fitting on the bench.) Curl up as before.

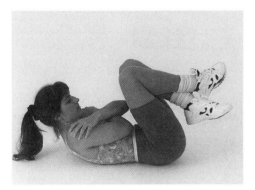

FIGURE 7.31

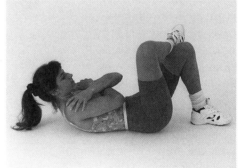

FIGURE 7.32

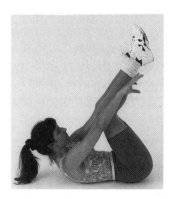

FIGURE 7.33

LOWER ABDOMEN
Muscle worked: rectus abdominis

Position 1

Lie flat on the back with the legs bent so that the knees are near the chest but the feet are extended upward.

Action   Try to lift the hips toward the ceiling while moving the knees toward the chest (Figure 7.34). (Try not to roll or use momentum—make the lower abdominals work.) Relax hips to floor. This exercise is often called a reverse curl.

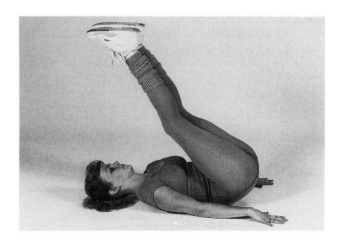

FIGURE 7.34
Reverse curl.

Position 2

Sit on the floor with the legs extended to the front. Lean back on the elbows. Roll the pelvis under so that the lower back is on the floor. (Some people are more comfortable lying flat and supporting the hips with the hands.)

Action Bicycle the legs (Figure 7.35). If fatigue causes the lower back to lift off the floor, bicycle with just one leg.

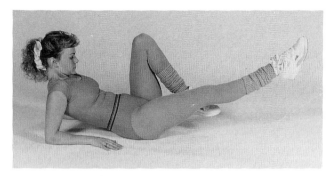

FIGURE 7.35

SIDES OF ABDOMEN
Muscles worked: obliques

Position 1

Assume curl-up position.

Action Twist the torso to one side before curling up (Figure 7.36a). If the hands are by the head in a more advanced position, leave one elbow on or near the floor while twisting and lifting with the opposite side of the body (Figure 7.36b). Curl-ups may be performed in a series to one side or alternating sides.

Variations

1. Alternately extend one leg out and hold it off the floor and bend the other leg into the chest. As the legs change position, twist and curl, bringing the left elbow to the right leg or the right elbow to the left leg. (Figure 7.37 shows this with an advanced arm position.)

2. Lay the knees over to one side, placing the body in a twisted position. Curl up. (Figure 7.38 shows an advanced arm position.)

Position 2

Lie flat on back with legs bent and one foot off the floor.

Action With bent legs, lay the left knee down to the left and then bring it back up to center (Figure 7.39). Repeat with the right knee to the right side. This exercise will also work the inner thigh.

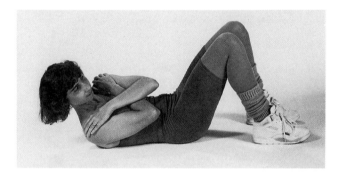

FIGURE 7.36a

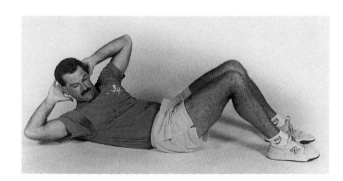

FIGURE 7.36b Advanced arm position.

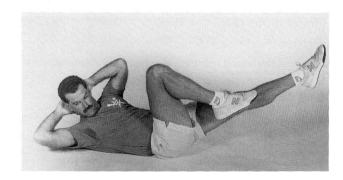

FIGURE 7.37 Advanced arm position.

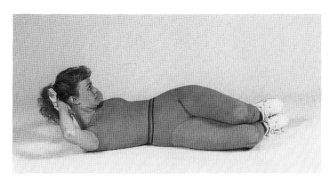

FIGURE 7.38 Advanced arm position.

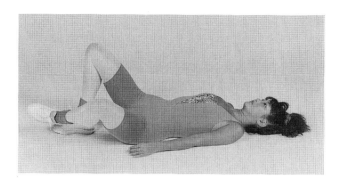

FIGURE 7.39

Back

Throughout this text are technique pointers to help prevent back injury. Here are three exercises that can help strengthen your back. Always work with good postural alignment and always stop if you feel pain.

SHOULDERS AND UPPER BACK
Muscle worked: trapezius

Position

Stand with good posture.

Action   Shrug the shoulders up, hold for 3 to 5 seconds, then relax down (Figure 7.40).

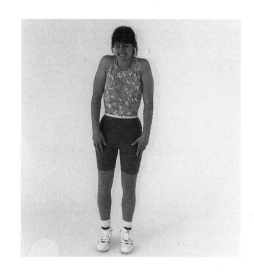

FIGURE 7.40

UPPER BACK
Muscles worked: trapezius, rhomboids

Position

Stand with arms in front of the body parallel to the floor. (Figure 7.41a).

Action   Draw the elbows back, keeping the arms parallel to the floor. Initiate the movement with the muscles in the back. Try to pinch the shoulder blades together (Figure 7.41b). Relax shoulders and arms.

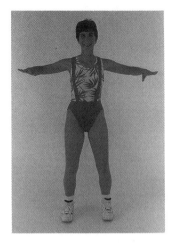

FIGURE 7.41a

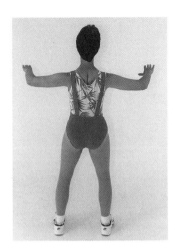

FIGURE 7.41b

BACK AND BUTTOCKS
Muscles worked: erector spinae, gluteals

Position

Lie prone with both arms extended overhead along the floor.

Action   Raise one arm and the opposite leg simultaneously. Keep both the arm and the leg straight. Hold for 5 to 10 seconds and then relax (Figure 7.42). If you experience any pain, discontinue this exercise.

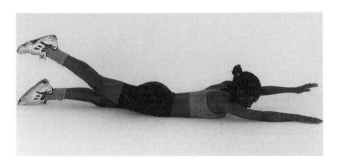

FIGURE 7.42

SUMMARY

Working muscles correctly will increase your rate of improvement. Be sure to isolate the muscle or muscle group you are trying to train. If your muscles begin to cramp during an exercise, stop and stretch them out. If the instructor and class are doing more of an exercise than you can do, perform one for every two they do. To gain fitness, overload by working until you feel mild discomfort, but never perform an exercise that causes pain. Finally, don't be afraid to modify exercises to make them safer and more comfortable for you.

KNOWLEDGE TIPS

1. Body toning exercises are primarily anaerobic.

2. Body toning exercises can improve both muscular strength and endurance.

3. You can make an exercise more difficult (intense) by changing position or by adding resistance in the form of weights or exercise bands.

4. Move at a moderate pace and maintain body control throughout the exercise.

5. Exercise both muscles of a muscle pair.

6. Use a curling motion during sit-up–type exercises.

7. Avoid exercises that strain the lower back.

8. If muscle cramping occurs, stop and stretch.

CHAPTER 8

Body Toning Using Bands, Weights, and Water

Body toning exercises can be made more difficult if participants increase the amount of resistance against which the muscles must move. This chapter discusses how exercise bands, weights, and water can be used to increase resistance.

A few safety considerations are crucial when you are increasing resistance to an exercise. You must maintain good body alignment and a full range of motion. As with any strength exercise, you should:

- Warm up thoroughly before beginning and work with controlled movements.

- Isolate the muscle you want to work, and keep all the other muscles relaxed unless you are using them to stabilize your body position.

- Avoid locking your joints.

- Balance your workout to prevent muscle soreness and to maintain a balance between the strength of the agonist and that of the antagonists.

- Be sure to breathe during the exercises. Breathe out during the work phase and breathe in as you relax.

- Be sure to stop if at any time you feel pain, because this is your body's way of telling you that you have imposed too much of an overload.

As long as you follow these basic rules, you can add weights and bands to all the exercises in Chapter 7 except the neck exercises and the back lift from the prone position. For example, the arm curl can be

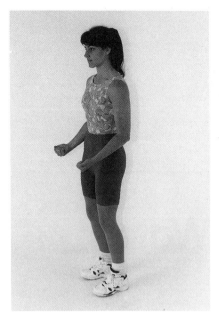

FIGURE 8.1a

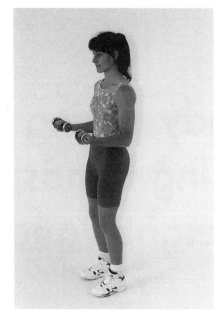

FIGURE 8.1b

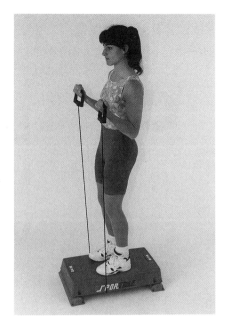

FIGURE 8.1c

performed by itself (Figure 8.1a), with hand-held weights (Figure 8.1b), or with a cable-style exercise band (Figure 8.1c). The basic curl technique and body alignment does not change. In this chapter, a variety of band exercises are pictured to help you learn how to wrap or hold the band. Pictures using weights are not included since they would be the same as the pictures in Chapter 7 with the exception of a weight held in the hand or wrapped around an ankle or wrist.

EXERCISE BANDS

Bands can be surgical tubing, cables with handles, heavy-duty large office-type rubber bands, or sheets of rubber 5 to 6 inches wide resembling strips of inner tubes. The latter are produced commercially for aerobics classes and therapeutic clinics under several names such as Dyna-bands and Therabands. They usually come in several colors, each color representing the amount of resistance: light, medium, or heavy. If you choose to use a band, take off any jewelry that may cut into the band. (You can wear weight-lifting or bicycling gloves to take the pressure off your hands and to cover jewelry you do not want to remove.) The commercially made bands that resemble office rubber bands come in several thick-

nesses; thin bands are less resistive than thick bands. Using the recommended range of 8 to 12 repetitions, you should change to a thicker or more resistant band when you can easily perform 12 repetitions and try a thinner or less resistant band if you can't do at least 8 repetitions. You may have to reduce band difficulty further if your goal is more endurance oriented and you intend to do more than 12 repetitions.

If you have high blood pressure or have suffered a cumulative trauma disorder such as carpal tunnel syndrome, check with a physician before starting an exercise band program. If you suffer knee problems, always work with the band above your knees. If you have other joint problems, avoid heavy resistance training and check with your physician before using exercise bands. Bands may pull on leg hair, so socks, tights, or sweat pants are recommended.

The following band exercises are a representative sample of what can be done with bands. Note that for every flexion exercise there is also an extension exercise. The exercises are described and pictured for one side only. Be sure to work both the right and the left side. Start with one set (of 8 to 12 repetitions) and build up to between two and five sets. For more exercises and information on exercise bands, look for books written by qualified experts.

ARM CURL (FLEXION)
Muscles worked: biceps

Position

Stand on one end of band. With hand on same side of body as the foot, grasp or wrap band around hand. The arm starts in an extended relaxed position.

Action Flex the arm, bringing the palm toward the shoulder (Figure 8.2). Slowly lower the hand.

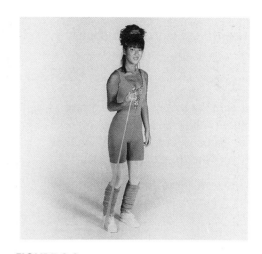

FIGURE 8.2

ARM EXTENSION
Muscles worked: triceps

Position

Stand with knees slightly bent. Grasp middle of band with one hand and hold it against chest next to opposite shoulder. Grasp one or both of the ends with other hand. The lower hand should be directly below upper hand.

Action Pull down with the bottom hand until the arm is extended (Figure 8.3). Keep the elbow by the body throughout the motion. (The lower hand may have to grasp higher on the band to get a full range of motion.) Slowly flex (relax) the arm.

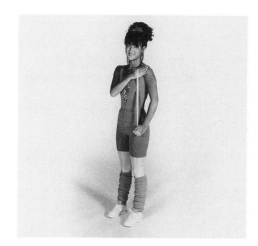

FIGURE 8.3

CHEST PRESS
Muscles worked: pectorals

Position

Stand with knees slightly flexed. Hold one end of the band in each hand with the band running across the shoulder blades and under the arms.

Action Extend both arms forward (Figure 8.4a). Slowly flex (relax) the arms.

Variation Perform the same exercise lying down on a bench with band running under bench. Keep knees bent and low back flat (Figure 8.4b).

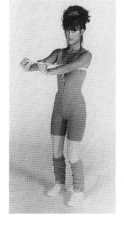

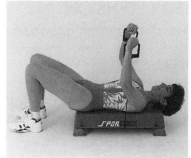

FIGURE 8.4b

FIGURE 8.4a

SEATED ROW
Muscles worked: trapezius, rhomboids (upper back)

Position

Sit on the floor with the legs extended forward. (If this position is uncomfortable, the knees may be bent.) Hold one end of the band with each hand with the band running across the soles of the shoes.

Action Pull both hands back toward the armpits (Figure 8.5). Squeeze the shoulder blades together at the same time. Slowly extend the arms and relax the back.

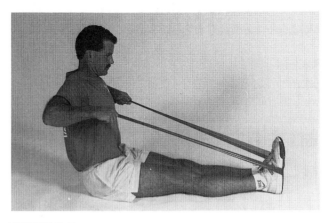

FIGURE 8.5

LEG CURL (FLEXION)
Muscles worked: hamstrings

Position

Lie prone. Band is tied around both ankles, leaving about an inch between ankles. Hands can be under the chin or under the hips.

Action Bend one leg up toward the buttocks while holding the other leg down (Figure 8.6a). The leg should be flexed until the sole of the foot is directed at the ceiling (90 degrees). Slowly lower the leg.

Variation For a more advanced exercise, stand and bend one leg up toward the buttocks, flexing the bent knee to 90 degrees (Figure 8.6b). Slowly lower the leg.

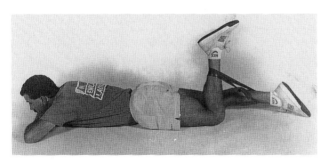

FIGURE 8.6a

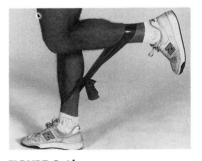

FIGURE 8.6b

LEG EXTENSION
Muscles worked: quadriceps

Position

Sit with knees bent and feet flat on the floor. Lean back on the elbows. Band is tied around both ankles, leaving about an inch between ankles.

Action Extend one leg forward (Figure 8.7). Slowly lower the leg.

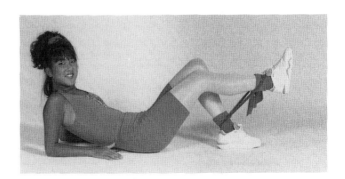

FIGURE 8.7

SIDE STEP
Muscles worked: abductors (outer thigh)

Position

Stand with feet together and knees slightly flexed. Band is tied and placed above the knees (beginner), below the knees (intermediate), or around the ankles (advanced).

Action Step to one side, maintaining knee bend. Slowly slide in the opposite foot (Figure 8.8a). Bands can also be used in a side-lying leg lift (Figure 8.8b).

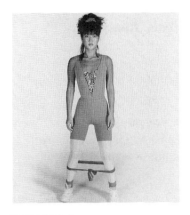

FIGURE 8.8a

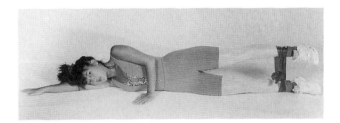

FIGURE 8.8b

INNER THIGH LIFT
Muscles worked: adductors

Position

Lie on one side with top leg bent and knee placed on the floor in front of the body. Band is tied around both ankles with about an inch between ankles.

Action Lift the bottom leg up toward the ceiling (Figure 8.9). Slowly lower the leg to the floor.

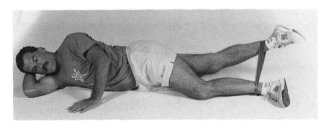

FIGURE 8.9

HIP AND TRUNK CURL (FLEXION)
Muscles worked: hip flexors (quadriceps, iliopsoas), abdominals

Position

Lie on back, with knees bent toward chest. Band is tied around legs just above knees. Hands are placed inside the band loop, with palms facing feet.

Action Curl knees toward chest while simultaneously holding the band in position or pushing it away. The upper body can also be curled toward knees (Figure 8.10). Slowly uncurl legs and upper body.

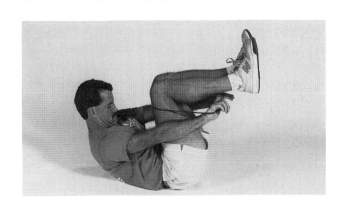

FIGURE 8.10

HIP EXTENSION
Muscles worked: gluteals, hamstrings

Position
Lie prone. Band is tied around both ankles, leaving about an inch between.

Action   Keeping the legs straight, lift up one leg with the heel leading. Keep both hips in contact with the floor (Figure 8.11). Slowly lower the leg.

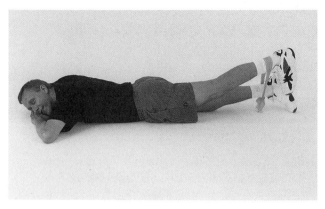

FIGURE 8.11

LAT PULL-DOWN
Muscle worked: latissimus dorsi

Position
Stand with knees slightly bent. Band is held overhead in both hands, palms forward, with the anchor hand (left) centered above and behind the head and the anchor arm elbow slightly bent.

Action   Pull the band down and to the side by drawing the working elbow (right) down toward the waist (Figure 8.12). Slowly relax the working arm and allow it to return to its original position.

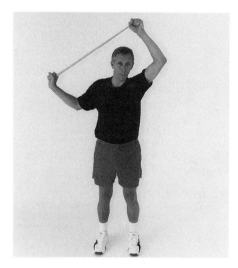

FIGURE 8.12

ANKLE FLEXION
Muscle worked: anterior tibialis

Position
Sit on the floor with knees bent in front of the body and hands supporting behind the buttocks. The band, tied snugly around both feet, runs across the top of the arch of the right foot and under the sole of the left foot.

Action   Flex the right foot—that is, draw the toes toward the shin (Figure 8.13). Slowly point (relax) the foot.

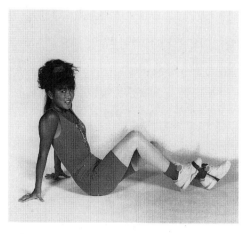

FIGURE 8.13

ANKLE EXTENSION
Muscles worked: gastrocnemius, soleus

Position

Sit on the floor with legs extended out in front. Hold one end of the band in each hand with the band running across the ball of one or both feet. The foot should be in a flexed position.

Action   Extend the foot by pointing the toes (Figure 8.14). Caution: Do not let the band slide off the foot. Slowly flex (relax) the foot.

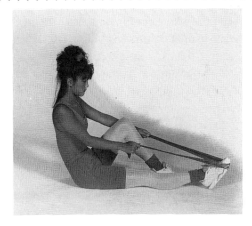

FIGURE 8.14

WEIGHTS

Only advanced students who do not have a history of joint problems (tendinitis, bursitis, arthritis, and others) should use weights. Hand-held, wrist, and ankle weights can all be used for body toning exercises. Weights should never be used during warm-up or cool-down activities.

You should add weight to an exercise only when the exercise is relatively easy to perform without weight. Start with small weight increases of 1/2 to 1 pound. When a weight is swung through the air, speed and momentum give it a force greater than its actual weight. (Think of the damage a wrecking ball can do when it is swung into a building.) The muscles, tendons, and ligaments around a joint have to stop the weight at the end of their range of motion. Too much weight, amplified by indiscriminate flinging of the arm or leg, can tear these tissues. Work with an appropriate amount of weight and always use controlled, fluid movements.

Weights come in three forms: hand-held, circular elastic, and wraparound. The advantages of hand-held weights are that they come in a wide variety of weights and that they are easy to control. The disadvantages are that people tend to grip them too tightly, causing irritation of the wrist tendons and that having to hold something in your hands may feel awkward. In addition, although hand-held weights can be used for lower-body strengthening, they must be used in lunge and squat exercises rather than leg-lift exercises. Elastic weights have the advantages of slipping onto the working limb (arm or leg), leaving the hands free for supporting the body, and allowing the exerciser to slide the weight up the limb to lighten the resistance, since weight closer to the center of the body is easier to lift. The disadvantage of elastic weights is that they may slide around and be annoying if they are too big. Wrist and ankle weights that wrap on with Velcro adjustable closures have the advantage of adjusting to limb size.

WATER

To move your body through water, you have to move the water that is in your way. Pushing or pulling against the water provides a resistance that can be used for strength and endurance conditioning. Out of the water, air resistance during body toning is minimal, but having to work against gravity is significant. In the pool you are more buoyant (lessening the effect of gravity), but the water offers 12 times more resistance to movement than does air.

You can increase water resistance using the following five methods. First, move the broadest body surface possible through the water. For example, moving a flat palm through the water creates more resistance than moving the edge of the hand through water. Moving a webbed glove or plastic barbell through the water similarly increases the amount of surface and therefore resistance. Second, increase the length of the resistance arm of a lever. The arms and legs of the body act like levers, and when the arm or leg is extended it meets more resistance going through the water than when it is bent. Third, exert more force against the water. Moving a body part through the water quickly (with more force) is harder than moving it slowly through the water. Fourth, change the direction of moving water. Sweeping water in one direction and then reversing directions forces your muscles to work harder as they fight the current. Finally, move as much water as possible. Once you get a block of water moving, momentum will keep it moving and your limb will get to rest a little. Instead of continuing to push right behind the block of moving water, change the position of your arm up or down and pick up a new block of water. Circular and undulating movement patterns move more water than do straight-line movements.

Body toning exercises performed in water are similar to those on land, but aqua body toning has two distinct advantages. The first is that resistance is applied in both directions of an exercise. As the leg sweeps out to the side in a leg lift, the outer thigh muscles work against the water. As the working leg is brought back in, the inner thigh works against the water. As long as equal force is applied in each direction, muscle balance is achieved. The second advantage is that people of all abilities can exercise together because it's simple to adjust the intensity of the exercise. For example, participants can perform a lower-body exercise of jumping off

the bottom of the pool by pushing off with a little or a lot of force. Grandparent and grandchild can do this together and both benefit! The intensity can also be adjusted in very small increments, unlike weights or bands where you jump to the next available resistance level. Most people find water aerobics to be fun and easy on their bodies. To learn more, consider taking a course or purchasing a good water (aqua) aerobics book.

SUMMARY

You can increase your muscular strength and endurance by progressively overloading. One way to achieve an overload is to increase the resistance against which the muscles work. You can increase resistance by adding weights or exercise bands to body toning exercises or by performing the exercises in water.

KNOWLEDGE TIPS

1. Resistance can be increased through the use of exercise bands and weights or by performing exercises in water.

2. Only individuals exercising at intermediate to advanced levels who find the basic exercises easy and who have very good exercise technique should use weights and exercise bands.

3. Individuals with joint injury, high blood pressure, heart disease, or orthopedic problems should not use weights or bands without consulting their physician.

4. Breathe out during the work phase and in during the relaxation phase.

5. Maintain good body alignment and move with control through a full range of motion.

6. Start with low levels of resistance and use progressive overloads to achieve higher levels of fitness.

7. Gradually overload by increasing resistance or repetitions (or sets), but not both in one day.

8. Make aqua exercises more difficult by presenting the broadest body surface to the water, extending a limb, moving through water with greater force, changing the direction of moving water, and moving more blocks of water.

CHAPTER 9

Exercises to Avoid

Someone once said that a weed is a flower out of place. So it is in exercise; some exercises are weeds when they appear in aerobic dance exercise yet are flowers in specific sports settings. The hurdler's stretch (Figures 9.1a and 9.1b) is a perfect example. People who compete in the hurdle run at track meets need to stretch out in this position, since it is the exact position they use to go over the hurdle. It is not, however, a good exercise for the general public because it places a considerable amount of torque on the knee. Hurdlers try to limit use of this stretch for the same reason.

Hyperextension exercises are another good example. Gymnasts often have to arch their back to perform tumbling stunts and to accent dance movements. Yet for the average person, these positions place the back, particularly the vertebral discs, in a very stressful position.

The rest of this brief chapter illustrates some stretching positions and strengthening exercises not recommended for the general public along with captions explaining why they are not recommended. This list is not comprehensive; it simply includes some of the most commonly used stressful exercises. If you keep in mind some of the technique tips presented in Chapters 7 and 8, you will probably be able to evaluate new exercises and determine whether they are good for you. When in doubt, be sure to ask your instructor.

As you look at these exercises, try to figure out how to fix them, or what exercises you could substitute to achieve the same stretch or strengthening effect. Check your answers against the list at the end of this chapter.

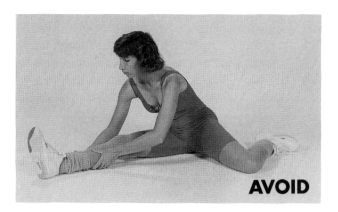

FIGURE 9.1a
Stretching forward in the hurdler's stretch stresses the knee ligaments.

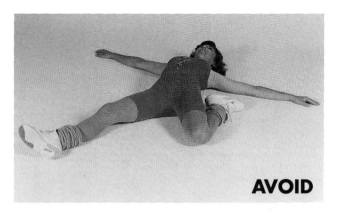

FIGURE 9.1b
Leaning back in the hurdler's position stresses knee ligaments and the lower back.

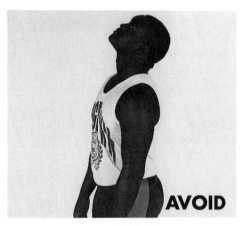

FIGURE 9.2
Hyperextending the neck stresses the cervical vertebrae.

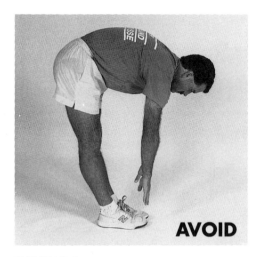

FIGURE 9.3
The straight-leg toe touch places stress on the ligaments in the lower back region.

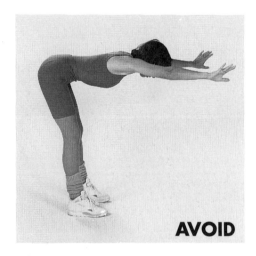

FIGURE 9.4
The flat back position stresses the muscles and ligaments in the lower back region.

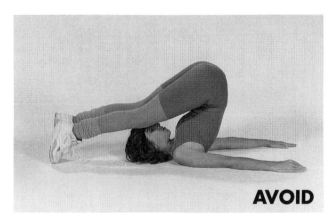

FIGURE 9.5
The plow position puts the weight of the entire body on the cervical vertebrae. It is very stressful to the spine.

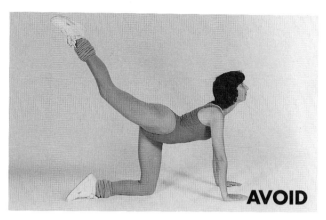

FIGURE 9.6
Kicking too high in the all-fours position causes the back to arch. This can be stressful to the spine.

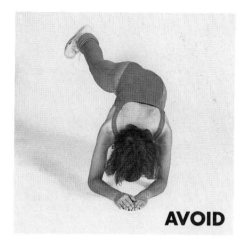

FIGURE 9.7
When the working leg is lifted out to the side instead of directly upward, the body's weight has to shift away from the leg for balance. This poor alignment can stress the back as well as interfere with the toning effect of the exercise.

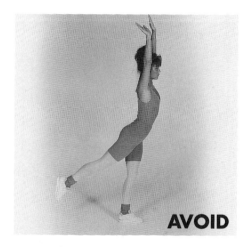

FIGURE 9.8
Kicking too high to the back accompanied with overhead arms that are pressing the upper trunk back results in a hyperextended back. This can be stressful to the spine.

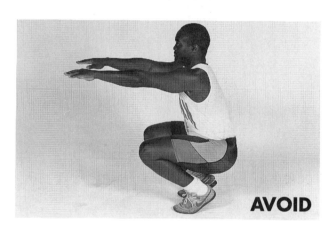

FIGURE 9.9
Deep knee bends place stress on knee ligaments.

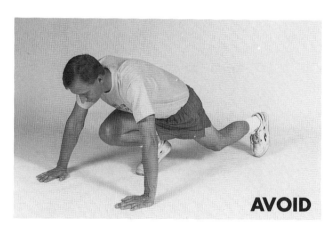

FIGURE 9.10
When the knee is pushed beyond the instep, pressure is placed on knee ligaments.

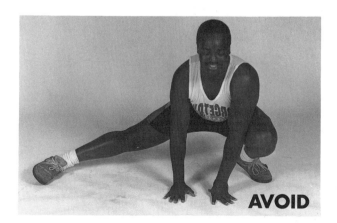

FIGURE 9.11
Again the knee extends beyond the instep, so stress is placed on knee ligaments.

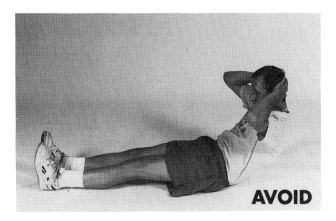

FIGURE 9.12
Straight-leg sit-ups place stress on the lower back and emphasize hip flexor strengthening, not abdominal strengthening. Placing the hands behind the head and pulling forward also stresses the cervical vertebrae.

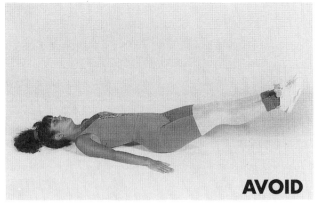

FIGURE 9.13
The weight of both legs is often more than the abdominals can handle. The result is stress on the lower back area.

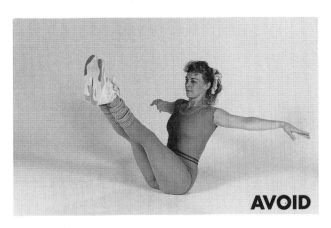

FIGURE 9.14
The V-seat position is another form of a double leg lift, stressing the lower back area.

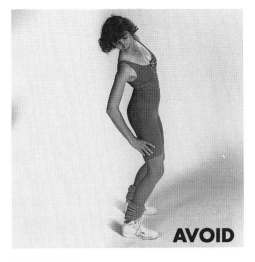

FIGURE 9.15
Poor alignment, pelvis rotated forward, when stretching to the side results in an arched back position and stress on the spine.

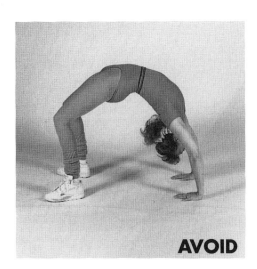

FIGURE 9.16
Hyperextension of the back is stressful to the spine.

SUMMARY

There is more than one way to stretch and strengthen your muscles. Select exercises that feel good to you. If the class is performing an exercise that you know will hurt your body, don't do it; modify the exercise or perform a different one. I have seen too many people give in to peer pressure. Instead of doing the "right thing" they have found it more important to look like the rest of the class. Be an individual and do the exercises that are right for you.

KNOWLEDGE TIPS

1. Some exercises are appropriate in sports settings and inappropriate in health-related fitness settings.

2. Avoid exercises that require you to lift both legs at the same time.

3. Avoid exercises and positions that strain joints.

4. Always work with good alignment.

SUGGESTIONS FOR MODIFYING OR CORRECTING THE EXERCISES TO AVOID

9.1a   Bend the knee, keeping the foot in front of the body near the inner thigh, page 40.

9.1b   Perform a standing or lying quadriceps stretch, page 37.

9.2   Perform head stretches to the front and sides and neck glides, page 34.

9.3   Bend both knees; better yet, stretch one leg at a time by extending it forward and bending toward it, page 39.

9.4   Bend both knees and alternately round and relax the back, page 36.

9.5   Two exercises can replace this: (1) head flexion (upper back can be rounded during this exercise), page 34; (2) a shoulder stretch, page 35.

9.6   Drop down on the forearms and bring the leg down until it is in line with the back, pages 65–66.

9.7   Bring the leg into center alignment, page 66.

9.8   Move the arms forward or down so that a straighter back alignment may be retained. Contract abdominals to support the back.

9.9   Flex knees only to 90 degrees, page 68.

9.10   Place the foot under the knee, page 40.

9.11   Place the foot under the knee, page 39.

9.12   Bend both knees and place the arms so that they don't pull on the neck, page 72 and 73.

9.13   Replace with single leg raises, reverse curls, or bicycling, pages 65, 73, and 74.

9.14   Same as 9.13.

9.15   Pull in abdominals and bend directly to the side; look forward to prevent twisting, page 36.

9.16   Perform back stretches in the prone position, page 42.

CHAPTER 10

The Benefits of Aerobic Dance Exercise

Some people would have you believe that all exercise does is make you sweaty, mess up your hair, take time out of your day, and produce a pile of dirty laundry. These people are making excuses for not being active: Millions of other people are physically active and rave about exercise.

Why do they rave? Maybe because they know that three to five hours a week of endurance training such as aerobic dance exercise can help prolong life, reduce the risk of heart disease, lower blood cholesterol, reduce weight and stress levels, improve self-image, tone and strengthen muscles, and improve flexibility. Or . . . maybe because they know exercise is a fun way to get fit and meet other people. There are a lot of good reasons to exercise. Combined with other healthy life-style habits, exercise can make you look and feel your very best.

This chapter is about reasons for exercising. It is about knowing how the body works and how exercise works on the body. Why should you know these things? Because they will help you take responsibility for your own health. You can choose the benefits that are important to you and make sure that the exercises that result in those benefits are included in your exercise program. With a basic understanding of exercise physiology you can talk with professionals on a more knowledgeable level, ask intelligent questions, and evaluate the quality of instruction you are receiving.

Somehow knowing the why of things makes doing them more worthwhile. As you tangle up your feet on a new aerobic step or struggle with a new overload, think about how strong your heart is getting, how much easier daily chores are with your newfound strength, and how fat is disappearing and nicely toned muscles are developing. Fill your head with positive thoughts, and you'll get through even the most sluggish days and feel better for it.

The human body is intricately engineered and fantastically coordinated. At this very moment, inside you, millions of chemical reactions are occurring, brain signals are flying along nerve pathways, muscles are contracting and relaxing to maintain your posture against gravity, food is being digested and converted to energy, and all these things and many more are happening simultaneously, routinely, and without conscious thought. Each of the systems in your body (cardiovascular, muscular, respiratory, and others) is influenced by exercise. Each system is affected in a manner specific to the kind of exercise performed. Aerobic dance exercise emphasizes improvement of the cardiovascular, respiratory, and muscular systems.

At rest, the body is in a state of balance called **homeostasis** in which energy is being produced at the same rate that it is being used. When you begin to exercise, your body uses energy faster than it is being produced. In an attempt to restore homeostasis, you breathe faster, your heart rate increases, your energy production increases, and you sweat more to dissipate heat. All these changes help you establish homeostasis at a higher level of energy production and utilization. When you stop exercising, the energy output decreases and your body adjusts once again. The changes involved in maintaining homeostasis are called short-term or acute adaptations.

Anything that disturbs homeostasis and causes the body to make changes is called a stressor. Exercise is a stressor. When the body is stressed repeatedly over time, long-term or chronic adaptations take place. The right amount of stress causes healthy changes. Too much stress results in unhealthy changes. For example, taking an aerobic dance–exercise class three to five times a week will tone your muscles. Taking two classes every day can overstress the muscles and lead to an injury. In the previous chapters you have learned how to set up a program with the amount of stress needed to maximize your long-term benefits. This chapter examines the systems of the body most affected by participation in aerobic dance exercise and discusses the long-term benefits of exercise for each system.

. . . .
THE METABOLIC SYSTEMS

The metabolic systems, often referred to as the energy systems, convert food into energy. The food you eat is broken down through various chemical pathways with the purpose of producing **adenosine triphosphate** (ATP), which is a high-energy phosphate molecule. When ATP is split apart it releases energy that the cells in your body can use. Muscle cells use ATP to fuel contraction, and movement is possible as long as ATP is available. (Nonavailability of ATP results in rigor mortis.) It is extremely important, then, to have ways to resynthesize ATP when it has been broken down for energy.

There are two types of energy systems: aerobic and anaerobic. The type, intensity, and duration of activity you are engaged in determines how much energy is produced by each system. It is important to note that activities are not purely aerobic or anaerobic. When an activity is referred to as aerobic, that means the energy for movement is predominantly, but not exclusively, supplied by the aerobic system. When you perform exercises that emphasize the aerobic system, you get a different kind of conditioning than when you emphasize the anaerobic system. Familiarity with these systems can help you select activities that will lead toward your fitness goals.

The Anaerobic Systems

Anaerobic means "without oxygen." During short, intense bursts of activity, the body cannot meet the muscle cells' demand for oxygen. For this situation, the body is equipped with two energy-producing systems that are not dependent upon oxygen. These **anaerobic systems** are rapid sources of ATP for short periods of time. In a sense, the cells are making energy while they hold their breath.

The most rapid anaerobic system is called the **phosphagen system.** The phosphagen system consists of small amounts of high-energy phosphagens stored directly in the muscle cell. As ATP is broken down, the high-energy phosphagens build it back up. This stored energy is used to get you going right at the beginning of exercise, especially if you start into it quickly. It is also what makes you leap out of your seat when someone yells *fire!* The muscle can store only enough high-energy phosphagens to produce ATP for one to six seconds of activity. Training the phosphagen system is really only important if you are going to compete in sports such as weight lifting and sprinting; anaerobic glycolysis and the aerobic system are much more important to lifetime fitness. As the phosphagen system is depleted, a second anaerobic system (anaerobic glycolysis) takes over as the main energy producer.

Anaerobic glycolysis breaks down carbohydrate (glucose) without oxygen to produce ATP. Along with energy, **lactic acid** and heat are produced. If the anaerobic activity is intense enough, the lactic acid builds up, makes the muscle feel heavy, and produces a burn. The buildup of lactic acid is associated with muscle exhaustion. When you stop exercising or drop to a lower intensity, the concentration of lactic acid decreases. The excess heat is dissipated through sweat. You breathe hard after an anaerobic bout of exercise because your body requires oxygen to clear up the lactic acid and to return the cardiorespiratory system to homeostasis. Because of the role lactic acid plays, anaerobic glycolysis is often called the **lactic acid system**.

Activities that depend on the anaerobic system for energy are generally short, intense, and powerful. Predominantly anaerobic activities are usually less than a minute in duration. Sprints and strength-training exercises are examples of anaerobic exercises. Many exercises are partly anaerobic and partly aerobic. Anaerobic glycolysis plays a major role in intense activities that last one to three minutes. People who run four-minute miles, for example, must be in excellent anaerobic and aerobic shape.

A number of exercise benefits are associated with anaerobic training. The most important are cardiovascular fitness (through interval training) and muscular strength and endurance. Anaerobic training will also increase your tolerance of lactic acid, which will enable you to work out longer at high intensities.

The Aerobic System

The aerobic system is slower in its production of energy than the anaerobic systems, but it is capable of producing more energy per unit of food. **Aerobic** means "with oxygen." The **aerobic system** breaks down carbohydrate (**aerobic glycolysis**) and fat (**fatty acid oxidation**) in the presence of oxygen to produce ATP (that is, energy), carbon dioxide, water, and heat. Carbon dioxide is transported by the blood to the lungs and is exhaled out of the body. The heat and water are lost through sweat.

It is easiest for the body to metabolize carbohydrate, so that is the first source of fuel for the aerobic system. When the body is convinced that it will have to meet an elevated energy demand for a long period of time, it will conserve carbohydrate and use fat. It takes more energy to initiate the burning of fat than carbohydrate, but fat is a much richer source of energy. The burning of fat is called fatty acid oxidation. (You may also hear it called beta oxidation.)

Fatty acid oxidation has to be coaxed into operation. To benefit from this process you need to exercise for at least twenty minutes. If your goal is to burn fat it is better to exercise for a longer time at a moderate intensity than for a shorter time at a higher intensity.

Aerobic exercises are continuous, rhythmic activities using large-muscle groups. Swimming, cycling, brisk walking, cross-country skiing, and aerobic dancing are all aerobic activities. The many health benefits associated with aerobic conditioning are discussed in more detail in the discussion on the cardiovascular system. Cardiorespiratory endurance, weight management, and some muscle endurance are the primary benefits of aerobic training.

THE CARDIOVASCULAR SYSTEM

To understand the cardiovascular system better, picture it (heart, blood vessels, and blood) as an elaborate grocery delivery and garbage removal system. The blood loads oxygen at the lungs, travels down the roadways of the arteries, and delivers it to the doorstep of the cell. The cell takes in the oxygen and other nutrients it needs and unloads waste products such as carbon dioxide into the blood. The blood then travels back toward the heart through the veins, dumping the waste products off at the appropriate dump sites such as the lungs, liver, and kidneys. The heart is the pump that drives the whole system.

The speed of oxygen delivery and waste removal are controlled by the heart. When you start to exercise, your muscle cells call for more oxygen. Your heart picks up its pace so that oxygenated blood is moved to your cells more quickly. After exercise your heart rate declines rapidly for one minute and then declines more slowly as your body reestablishes homeostasis (balance). During recovery, by-products such as lactic acid are removed or converted into other chemical forms. The more efficient your cardiovascular system, the more quickly the heart rate returns to a resting value.

The average healthy heart has a resting heart rate of 70 to 80 beats per minute. The amount of blood the heart ejects with one beat is called the **stroke volume.** The **cardiac output** is the amount of blood pumped out of the heart in one minute. Increasing either the heart rate or the stroke volume will increase the cardiac output. When you exercise, both the stroke volume and the heart rate increase, but the heart rate increases much more dramatically. Stroke volume increases until about 40 percent of VO_2max; after that the increase in cardiac output is due to the heart rate. If the heart beats very fast, the stroke volume actually decreases because the chambers of the heart don't have enough time to completely fill.

Blood pressure is the pressure exerted by the blood against the walls of the arteries. When the heart is filling, the pressure in the arteries is fairly low. This is called the **diastolic pressure.** When the heart contracts, blood is forced out into the arteries, increasing the pressure of the blood against the arterial walls. This is called the **systolic pressure.** The body is infused with oxygen-rich blood during systole. Blood pressure is expressed as a fraction with systolic pressure on top and diastolic pressure on the bottom. Resting blood pressure readings below 140/90 are considered normal.

When you exercise, your blood pressure rises because your heart contracts more often and pushes higher volumes of blood into your arteries. Healthy arteries stretch and can handle the extra blood flow without any problem. Blood pressure stays in a healthy range even with the added stress of exercise. To appreciate the ability of the arteries, imagine an airport or train station with hallways that can expand at prime time to accommodate the extra travelers. Diseases that harden the arteries **(arteriosclerosis)** or cause plaque buildup, narrowing the arteries **(atherosclerosis),** cause the blood pressure to rise. Diseased arteries cannot withstand the same amount of stress as healthy arteries, so diseased arteries can severely limit your activity level.

Large arteries starting near the heart branch off into smaller and smaller arteries. The blood in the smallest arteries, called **capillaries,** delivers oxygen to the cells. The blood in the heart does not supply the heart with oxygen. Instead, small arteries that branch off the main artery near the heart take oxygen to the heart cells. These arteries are called **coronary arteries.** The heart is nourished with oxygen-rich blood during diastole through these coronary arteries.

Both aerobic and anaerobic exercise can improve cardiovascular fitness. However, to achieve cardiovascular fitness with anaerobic training, you must train at very high intensities. All-out efforts for short amounts of time are alternated with short rest periods. Many people find this kind of exercise difficult. In addition, it is too intense for beginners and older individuals. Aerobic dance exercise uses aerobic conditioning to achieve cardiovascular fitness. The more moderate intensity and continuous nature of aerobic conditioning seem to be more comfortable for most people. Since aerobic dance exercise uses aerobic conditioning to improve cardiovascular fitness, the benefits of cardiovascular training are discussed in terms of aerobic benefits.

Benefits of Exercising the Cardiovascular System

The heart muscle becomes stronger with exercise. Like the skeletal muscles, the cardiac (heart) muscle can improve in strength. It increases a little in thickness and contracts with greater force. The stroke volume also increases, which means the heart can pump more blood with each beat or the same amount of blood with fewer beats. As a result, the resting heart rate decreases. A few beats less per minute saves the heart a lot of beating over a lifetime.

The resting heart rate is influenced not only by the stroke volume but also by other efficiency improvements in the circulatory system. People who are highly trained aerobically may have resting heart rates as low as 45 beats per minute. These are exceptional athletes. Among aerobic dance–exercise veterans it is not uncommon to hear about resting heart rates in the 60s, 50s, and even 40s. Heredity also plays a role in establishing the resting heart rate. Some individuals who are not aerobically fit may have inherited a low resting heart rate. Similarly, some highly trained individuals have average (70–80 bpm) resting heart rates. But in general, as you train, your resting heart rate declines.

Exercise improves the ability of the cardiovascular system to deliver oxygen to the muscles. The ability of the blood to pick up and transport oxygen to the cells improves. The cells also improve in their ability to extract oxygen from the blood. The more oxygen you can supply your cells and the more efficient your muscle cells become at using it, the longer you can exercise.

A trained individual can exercise longer and with less fatigue than an untrained individual. Think of two people in the same aerobics class working out at the same pace. The one in better shape is working out at a lower percentage of her maximum heart rate or aerobic capacity. In addition, the fit individual will enter into fatty acid oxidation more quickly than the unfit person.

Aerobic exercise also causes an increase in the number and size of mitochondria. Think of mitochondria as power plants located in the muscle cells. All energy necessary for cell functioning during aerobic exercise is produced in the mitochondria. The mitochondria are more able to utilize fat as an energy source during exercise because the number of mitochondrial enzymes increases.

Imagine, for a moment, a city with only one main freeway. As rush hour hits, the freeway becomes congested. When an accident occurs it stops traffic. Some cars head for the surface streets, but if these streets are inadequate, they too quickly get congested. However, if a city has a well-developed highway system and plenty of surface streets, traffic moves with ease even during peak hours.

Exercise increases the number of capillaries (surface streets), and through cholesterol regulation, it helps keep the arteries (highways) clear. An increase in the number of capillaries means better oxygen/carbon dioxide exchange at the cellular level. It also means that when an artery becomes blocked, blood flow can be diverted to other healthy branches. This ability to divert blood flow is extremely important in the coronary network of arteries. Coronary circulation improves with endurance exercise: This helps prevent heart attacks.

Aerobic exercise increases the level of HDL (high-density lipoproteins) in your blood. HDL helps carry fat out of the bloodstream, which helps prevent it from forming plaque along the arterial walls. Plaque formation narrows arteries, thus restricting blood flow, raising blood pressure, and limiting stress-free activity. See the discussion on cholesterol in Chapter 11.

Evidence also indicates that exercise helps minimize the risk of having a heart attack and improves your chances of survival if you do have one. Improved cardiovascular fitness is also believed to reduce stress-induced tension and to provide a sense of well-being.

THE RESPIRATORY SYSTEM

The respiratory system and the cardiovascular system work together to deliver oxygen to the cells. Endurance exercise increases the amount of air you can breathe into your lungs. Each red blood cell has the capacity to carry one molecule of oxygen, yet blood is almost never 100 percent saturated. The blood moves by the lungs too quickly to load all the red blood cells with oxygen. Endurance training, however, can improve the blood's ability to load and unload oxygen.

THE SKELETAL SYSTEM

Each of the 206 bones in the human skeleton is a living entity. The bones you see when you look at a skeleton are dead. They give you a good idea of the shape and placement of living bones, but they do not represent live bone any more than the steak on your plate represents the living flesh of a cow. Living bones generate new bone tissue and repair and maintain healthy bone structure. Blood circulates through the bone tissue delivering nutrients.

Benefits of Exercising the Skeletal System

When you are active (walking, jumping, aerobic dancing, etc.), you stress your bones. The bones adapt by becoming stronger and more dense. Many researchers believe that exercise helps prevent osteoporosis, a disease that causes bones to become porous and brittle.

Osteoporosis is most common among postmenopausal women and is often the cause of broken hips or crushed vertebrae in elderly women. Proper nutritional care, in particular sufficient calcium intake, also plays an important role in preventing osteoporosis.

Although insufficient stress can cause bone weakening, too much stress can misshape, misalign, and even fracture a bone. The most common aerobic dance injury in this category is the lower leg stress fracture, which can be very painful and is so thin that it is difficult to observe on an X-ray. Set reasonable levels of intensity, duration, and frequency, and buy good shoes to help prevent such an injury.

Good posture is vital for maintaining proper bone alignment. If you walk around with your shoulders forward, eventually your spine and shoulder girdle bones will adjust to that posture, making it impossible to stand straight. Poor posture also leads to muscular problems, aches, and pains. Think of posture and alignment throughout your aerobics class as well as during the day. A tip from my mother: Stand tall every time you walk through a door. If you do not develop good posture, at least you will always make a grand entrance!

THE MUSCULAR SYSTEM

The three kinds of muscle are skeletal (striated), cardiac, and smooth. Skeletal muscles, attached to the bones by tendons, make it possible for us to move around; the heart is composed of cardiac muscle; and smooth muscle constitutes internal organs. Both cardiac and smooth muscle are involuntary, which means they contract without conscious thought. You don't have to think about making your stomach wall contract during digestion, nor do you command your heart to beat. Skeletal muscles are voluntary: you make conscious decisions as to how and when you want to move them. (Reflex movements of the skeletal muscles are the exception. During a reflex action, orders come from the spinal cord rather than the higher brain centers. The result is a very fast reaction that you don't consciously initiate.) Aerobic dance exercise develops both the cardiac and the skeletal muscles.

Muscles can only pull, not push; thus, they are paired together. One muscle pulls one way, the other muscle pulls the opposite way. When one is pulling, the other relaxes and stretches. The one doing the pulling is called the agonist; the one stretching is called the antagonist. When Popeye flexes his biceps, his lower arm is pulled closer to his upper arm. When he flexes his triceps (back of the upper arm), it pulls in the opposite direction, and his arm straightens out. When the biceps are working, the triceps are able to stretch and relax, and when the triceps are working, the biceps are able to stretch and relax.

When exercising muscles, it is important to work the muscle pairs equally. This way each stretches out the other, and strength balances are maintained. If you run on your toes throughout the aerobics section of a class, you have flexed (worked) your calf muscles the entire time. Stiffness will occur, and muscle imbalance may eventually lead to injury. Foot flexion exercises will work the muscles paired with the calf and allow the calf muscles to stretch. Because of this pairing, you can relieve a cramp in one muscle by flexing the opposite muscle: Relieve calf cramps by flexing the foot, arch cramps by lifting up on the toes.

Don't confuse working a muscle with the pull of gravity or with the use of an eccentric (or negative) contraction. If you flex your arm using the biceps and then let it fall straight down, you are using gravity, not the triceps, to do the work. When you lower your arm slowly, the biceps are working in what is known as an eccentric contraction. An **eccentric contraction** is the controlled lengthening of a contracted muscle. You are using an eccentric contraction when you slowly lower a heavy box. Again, the triceps are not working. The opposite of an eccentric contraction is a concentric contraction. During a **concentric contraction,** the muscle is shortening. When you flex your arms, the biceps are doing a concentric contraction; they are shortening. Whether you are using concentric or eccentric contractions, you always want to move with control.

Muscles are composed of fibers. The power or strength of a contraction depends on how many muscle fibers are recruited by the nervous system. If you are doing something that takes all your strength, then most of the muscle fibers will contract at one time. If you are relaxing after class, only the fibers needed to maintain muscle tonus are used. Muscle tonus is the amount of tension needed in the muscle. During relaxation only enough tension to maintain posture would be required.

Muscle spindles are specialized fibers that have stretch receptors. These spindles are responsible for the **stretch reflex.** When the muscle spindle's receptors are stretched suddenly, they send a signal to the spinal cord. The spinal cord sends back a message telling the surrounding muscle fibers to contract. The knee-jerk reflex is an example of this. When the doctor taps with a rubber hammer just below the knee, the patellar tendon, which attaches the thigh muscle to the bone, is suddenly stretched. The muscle spindles in the tendon react, the thigh muscle contracts, and the foot kicks.

Ballistic (bounce) stretching triggers the stretch reflex. Instead of relaxing and lengthening, the muscle gets the signal to contract. Proper static stretching does not excite the stretch receptors, so the muscle is able to relax and comfortably lengthen. Despite the stretch reflex, careful ballistic stretching can result in increased flexibility. However, it also carries a higher risk of tissue damage and muscle soreness than static stretching does.

Another kind of receptor, the Golgi tendon organ, sits among the muscle fibers. Golgi tendon organs have high thresholds for tension, but if tension becomes too great during a muscle contraction, they alert the brain to send a back-off message to the muscles. The back-off or relax message actually stays in effect for a short while after the contraction is stopped. In PNF (proprioceptive neuromuscular facilitation) stretching, the response of the Golgi tendon organs is purposefully elicited through an isometric contraction lasting 6 to 10 seconds. The muscle is stretched immediately after this contraction to take advantage of the relaxation phase induced by the Golgi tendon organ.

When the nervous system instructs a muscle to contract, it also alerts the antagonist (paired muscle) to relax. This is called reciprocal innervation. When you are trying to stretch a muscle you can use reciprocal innervation by consciously contracting the opposing muscle. This is called antagonist stretching. For example, if you wish to stretch your hamstring muscles, you can help them relax and lengthen by contracting your quadriceps muscles.

Benefits of Exercising the Muscular System

Muscles can improve in strength, endurance, and flexibility. The body toning exercises used in aerobic dance–exercise classes generally emphasize muscular endurance, but increases in strength can also occur, especially when exercise bands and weights are used. Flexibility is developed during the stretching segments of the class.

When muscles increase in strength, they may or may not **hypertrophy,** increase in size. Hypertrophy occurs only when enough of the hormone testosterone is present. This hormone is present in men in much larger amounts than in women. Interestingly, some muscle groups on an individual may hypertrophy more than others. For example, some men may have large shoulders and relatively small chests, even though they have worked on building strength in both areas.

Women do not usually have very much of this hormone, so they generally increase in strength without increasing in size. The muscle fibers tend to get stronger and pack down more densely, which results in an attractive toned and contoured look.

You may experience a temporary increase in muscle size while you are exercising due to the increased amount of blood being pumped to the working muscle. Some refer to this as being "pumped." The size of the muscle will begin to decrease when you stop exercising and will return to normal when increased blood flow is no longer needed. Because most women's muscles are relatively small, this increase in size is not very apparent. However, if you are going to take body measurements, be sure to do so before or well after exercising.

Anabolic steroids are drugs that can be taken to enhance strength gains, but they have dangerous side effects. They are most often associated with strength training for sports competitions. Today, many competitions, including the Olympics, consider anabolic steroid use illegal. Clearly these drugs do not belong in a health-related program.

Muscle endurance improves with exercise because the muscle cells become more effective at extracting oxygen and other nutrients from the blood and using them in the production of cellular energy. The oxygen goes into a structure inside the cell called the mitochondrion. The mitochondrion is often called the powerhouse of the cell, as it is inside these little factories that simple sugars (carbohydrates after digestion) are converted into cellular energy (ATP). The muscle adapts to endurance exercise by increasing the number of mitochondria. More mitochondria means more available ATP, which means more fuel for contractions. With more fuel available, movement (or exercise) can be sustained for a longer period of time. Think of all the ATP mitochondria have to produce for an hour of aerobics. Or for a marathon run!

Improving strength, endurance, and flexibility results in greater work efficiency, an improved ability to meet emergencies, and a decreased chance of lower back pain and injury.

OTHER SYSTEMS

Other systems affected by exercise include the nervous and reproductive systems. The nervous system is a fantastic communications system. Electrical impulses speed along nerve pathways delivering messages from the brain and spinal column. Aerobic conditioning improves the coordination of these transmissions, resulting in an ability to react with more speed, coordination, and

strength. Skill and coordination improve as you learn which muscles to stimulate and which to inhibit. A clear example is the difference between a beginning and an advanced swimmer. Beginners use practically every muscle in their bodies to stay afloat. The advanced swimmer uses only the necessary muscles. Beginning aerobics students experience a similar effect. They may start out feeling clumsy, but they quickly improve.

The effect of exercise on the reproductive system is difficult to study. Some researchers believe that exercise enhances sexual pleasure due to increased muscular strength and control. Two more serious issues regarding the effect of exercise on the reproductive system include the temporary loss of menstruation that sometimes occurs during high-level aerobic training and the effects of exercise on pregnancy. This loss of menstruation seems to be reversible, and a training regimen of lower intensity is recommended for women trying to conceive.

Guidelines for pregnancy and exercise have been published by the American College of Obstetricians and Gynecologists (ACOG). Exercise is healthy before, during, and after pregnancy for most women. A pregnant woman should consult her physician concerning the amount and type of exercise she can perform. There is some evidence that babies born to exercising mothers have fewer birth defects and that the mother's recovery time is faster. Women interested in exercising through pregnancy should start exercising before they become pregnant. For more information concerning exercise and pregnancy, see Chapter 12.

THE PSYCHOLOGICAL BENEFITS OF EXERCISE

Sport psychologists research the psychological effects of exercise. They have found that regular aerobic exercise increases the body's production of endorphins. Endorphins act like natural opiates, creating a sense of well-being. This feeling is often referred to as the runner's high. Regular exercise also acts as a release valve for stress: It helps relieve tension, lower anxiety, and lift depression. As people begin to look and feel better physically, they also tend to feel better about themselves mentally. An improved self-image can make you more confident and self-assured.

Unfortunately many people don't continue their exercise program long enough (six to eight weeks) to experience the invigorating natural highs. Adherence to exercise is a problem, but aerobic dance exercise has two characteristics that help people stick with it. First, people are more apt to continue doing something that involves music they like. Second, most people will continue in activities that involve social interactions. So the keys to experiencing the psychological benefits of exercise are to (1) get some of your friends to join you (2) encourage each other to keep exercising and (3) stick with it even if you are a little tired or depressed. You will feel better after the class!

SUMMARY

As you have seen, there are many good reasons to exercise. Although the cardiovascular, respiratory, and muscular systems improve the most with exercise, other systems of the body are also positively affected. As you exercise, try to picture all the fantastic changes that are being made in your body!

KNOWLEDGE TIPS

1. Exercise causes short-term or acute responses including an increased heart rate, increased systolic blood pressure, increased ventilation, and increased sweating.

2. Exercise causes long-term or chronic adaptations when it is done repeatedly over a period of time (see no. 5).

3. Aerobic exercises (continuous, rhythmic activities using large-muscle groups) use carbohydrate and fat for fuel.

4. Anaerobic exercises (intense activities of short duration) use carbohydrate for fuel.

5. The benefits of aerobically training the cardiovascular system include increased stroke volume, increased cardiac muscle strength, decreased resting heart rate, possible decreased blood pressure, increased aerobic capacity, increased coronary circulation, decreased risk of heart disease, increased work capacity, increased level of HDL, increased oxygen delivery to the muscles, increased numbers of capillaries, and an increased number of mitochondria.

6. Two benefits of training the respiratory system are increased lung capacity and an increased ability to deliver oxygen to the blood.

7. The benefits of training the muscular system include increased strength, increased muscular endurance, increased flexibility, increased work capacity, decreased risk of lower back pain, and decreased risk of injury.

8. Some benefits of training the skeletal system are increased bone density, maintenance of a good posture, and decreased risk of bone injury.

9. Other benefits of exercise include decreased mental tension, improved self-image, increased sense of well-being, regular digestion and excretion, improved sexual pleasure, and improved coordination and skill.

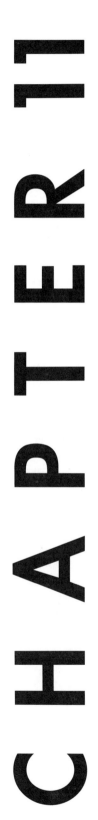

CHAPTER 11

Nutrition and Weight Control

Proper nutrition and exercise are two of the most valuable tools for developing and maintaining a healthy body. Used together, they are much more effective than either one alone. An exercise program without proper nutrition can leave you feeling run-down, depleted of energy, and without the building blocks for muscle and bone development. Similarly, a balanced diet without exercise doesn't result in muscle tone or aerobic efficiency. Put them together, and you not only get the positive effects of each one, you also experience combination benefits. This chapter starts with a review of basic nutritional information, then examines the combined effects of exercise and nutrition on weight control, and finally discredits some popular but false beliefs concerning dieting.

BASIC NUTRITIONAL INFORMATION

A car needs a variety of fluids to keep it running. You could say its nutritional requirements are gas for fuel, radiator fluid to keep the engine cool, and oil, transmission, and brake fluids to lubricate. If you fail to keep these fluids at appropriate levels, the car either runs poorly or doesn't run at all.

Your body, like a car, requires certain types and quantities of nutrients to function properly. The body's nutrients are chemicals that come from the digestion of food and drink. Your body needs about 50 different nutrients. These nutrients, organized into six categories, are referred to as the essential nutrients: carbohydrates, protein, fat, water, vitamins, and minerals.

Collectively, the six essential nutrients provide for the production of energy, the construction and maintenance of cells, and the regulation of body processes. Of these six, only three—carbohydrates, fat, and protein—provide energy for the body. When these nutrients are chemically broken down, energy is released. That energy is measured in kilocalories, which the general public calls **calories.** Fat provides almost twice as much energy (9 calories per gram) as carbohydrates and protein (4 calories per gram). Although no energy can be obtained from water, vitamins, or minerals, these nutrients play major roles in the many chemical processes of the body, including the processes that result in energy production.

Carbohydrates

Carbohydrates are the primary source of energy for the body. When sufficient amounts of carbohydrate and fat are available, protein is spared. Protein that is not used for energy production is used in the building and maintenance of tissues.

Carbohydrate foods (sugars and starches) are broken down into the simple sugar **glucose.** Glucose is absorbed into the blood and used by the cells. If it isn't used right away, glucose is stored in the muscles and liver as glycogen (long chains of glucose molecules). There are limits on how much glycogen can be stored, and when these limits are reached, additional glucose is converted into fat and stored as adipose tissue.

There are two kinds of carbohydrates: simple and complex. The natural sugars found in fruits and refined sugar are simple carbohydrates. Foods containing high amounts of refined sugars are easily digested and rapidly absorbed into the bloodstream. This occurs so quickly that they create a sudden surge in blood sugar, which triggers a release of insulin. In reaction to the high concentration of sugar in the blood, the insulin sweeps much of the sugar out of the blood. This, in turn, causes a sudden drop in blood sugar that leaves you feeling sluggish, tired, and often hungry. A sugary snack such as a candy bar is not a good way to get quick, lasting energy—that strategy generally backfires!

Foods that are composed of more complex sugars (starches), such as whole-grain cereals and vegetables, are sources of complex carbohydrates. For the most part, these foods are not easily digested so they are more slowly absorbed into the blood. This prevents quick rises and dips in the level of blood sugar. The resulting steady level of blood sugar helps you maintain your energy level and prevents you from feeling hungry between meals.

Sources of complex carbohydrates and natural sugars contain vitamins, minerals, and fiber, so eat them rather than refined sugars, which have no nutritional value. Carbohydrates should constitute 58 to 60 percent of your diet, where 48 percent of your diet should come from complex and natural sugar carbohydrate foods;

only 10 percent of your diet should consist of refined sugars, according to the United States Senate Select Committee on Nutrition and Human Needs.

Protein

Your body needs **protein** to build and repair body tissues, to make hemoglobin (which carries oxygen), to form antibodies (which fight infection), to produce enzymes and hormones, and, when necessary, to supply energy. When protein foods are digested, they are broken down into amino acids. There are nine amino acids that the body cannot manufacture. These nine are called essential amino acids. Foods that contain all the essential amino acids are called complete proteins; those that contain only some of the essential amino acids are called incomplete proteins. By eating two incomplete protein foods at the same meal, such as peanut butter and wheat bread, you can consume a full complement of amino acids. Lists of complete and incomplete proteins are available from the American Dairy Council. It is not necessary to take amino acid pills; it is easy to get all the protein you need in a normal diet. In fact, most Americans eat too much protein. When too much protein is consumed, the extra amino acids are converted to fat and stored. Only about 10 to 12 percent of a healthy adult's diet needs to be protein, even when a person is performing regular vigorous exercise. If you are a very active person, you need more calories but not a higher percentage of protein or fat. Increase all of your foods proportionally.

Fat

Fat is an essential part of every cell in your body. Complete removal of fat would result in death. (The absolute minimum for men is about 3 to 6 percent of body weight, for women about 8 to 12 percent.) Fat is an excellent source of concentrated energy. It also acts as insulation from the cold and carries the fat-soluble vitamins A, D, E, and K. Fat will provide energy for prolonged activities performed at low to moderate levels of intensity, but to do so, carbohydrate must also be present; it is often said that fat burns in a flame of carbohydrate.

The fat in foods is broken down into glycerol and fatty acids and put to use. Any extra fatty acids are converted and stored as adipose tissue. Fat should constitute no more than 30 percent of the diet. Unfortunately, the fat content in most Americans' diets is over 40 percent. You don't have to work hard at getting your required fat, since fat is hidden in so many foods. Red meats, cheeses, and fried foods are all high in fat.

Cholesterol is a fatty substance found in the blood and in body tissues. The body naturally synthesizes it because it is essential in the formation of bile salts, which are used in fat digestion. It is also an essential component of all cell membranes; therefore, it is found in every cell of the body. It is transported through the body by fat-protein particles called lipoproteins. Lipoproteins are named according to their density. The two major types of lipoproteins are **high-density lipoproteins (HDL)** and **low-density lipoproteins (LDL).** HDL picks up cholesterol from the cells and bloodstream and transports it to the liver where it is used to make the bile salts. When the bile salts are used for fat digestion, some of them are excreted, thus eliminating cholesterol from the body. HDL is sometimes called the garbage man of the blood since it picks up cholesterol and dumps it in the liver.

Cholesterol can be produced by the body or taken into the body in food. When the body has too much cholesterol, the LDL transporting cholesterol will give up its cholesterol to the walls of the arteries. As the fatty deposits (plaque) build up, the arteries become narrow and clogged. This condition, called atherosclerosis, is often accompanied by arteriosclerosis, a hardening of the arteries. Both of these can lead to **coronary heart disease,** a degenerative heart condition caused by the thickening and hardening of the coronary arteries. To prevent these dangerous diseases, people must control their cholesterol level. Plaque has been found in young adults and even in children; this disease does not start only in middle age.

The most effective way to control your cholesterol level is to eat a low-fat, low-cholesterol diet. Saturated fats, which are generally solid fats (animal fats, butter, cheese, and coconut and palm oils), are very high in cholesterol. Unsaturated fats, generally liquids or soft solids (corn oil, soybean oil, and margarine), are low in cholesterol. Try to eat unsaturated fats.

Both the total amount of cholesterol in the blood and the ratio of **total cholesterol** (TC) to HDL-carrying cholesterol (HDL-C) are good indicators of heart disease risk. A desirable level for total cholesterol is below 200 milligrams per deciliter. A TC/HDL-C ratio above 4.5 is associated with an elevated risk of heart disease, while a ratio below 3.5 indicates low risk. (To find out your cholesterol level, have a blood test done.) The ratio of cholesterol can be lowered by increasing the level of HDL, decreasing the level of LDL, or doing both. Aerobic exercise will increase the level of HDL. Eating a low-fat, low-cholesterol diet will decrease the level of LDL. A combination of diet and exercise is the best way to control your cholesterol level.

Water

Water, which constitutes 70 percent of the body's weight, is the solvent for digestion and for waste removal. Water represents the major component of blood and of the lubricant found in and around joints and organs. It also acts as a coolant as long as sweat is evaporating. You should drink six to eight 8-ounce glasses of water daily for normal activity.

As little as 2 to 3 percent dehydration affects physical performance. You can be this dehydrated and not even be thirsty. Furthermore, thirst can be quenched with small amounts of water when in fact your body may need much more. Be sure to stay well hydrated and don't trust your thirst as an indicator of dehydration.

During prolonged exercise, you should drink 1 to 1 1/2 cups of water before exercise (or competition), 1/2 cup every 10 to 15 minutes during exercise, and 2 cups for every pound lost after exercise. You may recall seeing water stations along running routes or water bottles at sports matches. Even though aerobic dance–exercise classes are usually shorter than sports practices, you should drink water before and after class and during a class in a hot environment.

You want to drink the fluid that will leave your stomach the most quickly and get out to the body where it is needed. Cold drinks (40°–50°F) leave the stomach more quickly than warm drinks. They also help cool you off. Even ice-cold water won't hurt you, although you should drink it slowly. Sugars (glucose, fructose, sucrose) in drinks slow down the rate at which the fluid leaves the stomach. Sport drinks should not exceed 1/2 teaspoon of sugar per 1/2 cup (2 to 2 1/2 grams per 100 ml). Unfortunately, most sport drinks have two to three times that amount of sugar. If you want to drink a sport drink, dilute it by one-half (1/2 cup sport drink plus 1/2 cup water). Soft drinks are not a good source of rapidly absorbed fluid. Fifteen minutes after drinking 12 ounces of a regular soft drink, 95 percent of it is still in your stomach. In addition, the carbonation can cause stomach bloating and upset. Fifteen minutes after drinking 12 ounces of water, only 30 percent of it is still in your stomach. Water is the most effective drink and also the least expensive.

Don't worry about replacing the electrolytes lost during an aerobics class. Sweat is really very diluted. The small amounts of minerals and electrolytes (including sodium [salt], potassium, and magnesium) that are lost through sweat can, in all but extreme cases, be replaced during your next regular meal. Avoid salt pills during exercise; they create a high salt concentration in the stomach that pulls water into the stomach for dilution and away from the body where it is needed. They may also cause stomach irritation and nausea.

Vitamins

Vitamins are organic compounds that are essential for the process of releasing energy from food. As a result, they help to control the growth of body tissues. Research evidence suggests that the lack of vitamins impairs physical performance, but no evidence has proven that large doses enhance performance. Large doses of the fat-soluble vitamins (A, D, E, and K) can accumulate over time and cause serious toxic effects. Excess water-soluble vitamins (B, C, and others) generally wash out of the body daily. However, megadose levels of intake of these vitamins can also result in serious problems. A balanced diet will usually provide all the vitamins you need. If you do supplement your diet, do so in moderation.

Minerals

Minerals are inorganic compounds that perform a variety of functions in the body. Some minerals, such as calcium, supply strength and rigidity to body structures such as bones and teeth. Adequate calcium intake is important to the prevention of osteoporosis (weakening of the bone). The mineral iron is critical to the formation of hemoglobin, which is the oxygen-carrying pigment in the red blood cell. Lack of iron can cause fatigue. Menstruating and athletic women require more iron than other women, and women in general need more iron than men. Other minerals are part of the composition of hormones such as insulin, while still others are involved in the regulatory functions of the body such as muscle contraction, nerve transmission, and blood clotting. A balanced diet will normally provide adequate amounts of all the minerals, but in some cases, iron and calcium supplements are needed.

THE FOOD PYRAMID

To ensure that you get all six essential nutrients, you should eat a balanced diet. The U. S. Department of Health and Human Services designed the food pyramid (Figure 11.1) as a guide for healthy eating. The shape of the pyramid suggests how much of each food group you should consume. Foods at the large base of the pyramid should make up the largest percentage of your diet. As the pyramid narrows, the number of recommended servings decreases.

Notice that the old four food groups have been redivided to form six food groups. Fats, oils, and sweets should be eaten sparingly because of the dangers of a high-fat and simple-sugar diet. The milk and meat groups require two to three servings, the fruit group two to four, and the vegetable group three to five servings. Table 11.1

FIGURE 11.1
The Food Guide Pyramid.

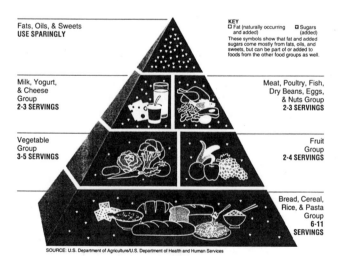

SOURCE: U.S. Department of Agriculture/U.S. Department of Health and Human Services

What Is the Food Guide Pyramid?

The Pyramid is an outline of what to eat each day. It's not a rigid prescription but a general guide that lets you choose a healthful diet that's right for you.

The Pyramid calls for eating a variety of foods to get the nutrients you need and at the same time the right amount of calories to maintain a healthy weight.

The Pyramid also focuses on fat because most American diets are too high in fat, especially saturated fat.

will give you an idea how much food represents a serving. The largest group, the bread and cereal group, requires six to eleven servings. Each of these groups has a range of servings. Your activity level, body size, and metabolism will all influence the number of calories you need to maintain a healthy body. If you are trying to gain weight, increase the number of servings proportionally to maintain your balance of 10 to 12 percent protein, 58 to 60 percent carbohydrate, and 30 percent fat.

In 1993, the Food and Drug Administration designed a new food label that is now required on almost all packaged foods. The label is designed to act as a guide to planning a healthy diet. The box on the following page shows an example of the new food label and offers some guidelines for interpreting the information contained on the new labels.

TABLE 11.1
Count as a serving.

Vegetables
1 cup of raw leafy greens, 1/2 cup of other kinds
1/2 cup of cooked dry beans or peas = vegetables or 1 ounce
    of meat

Fruit
1 medium apple, orange, or banana
1/2 cup of small or diced fruit
3/4 cup of juice

Grain Products
1 slice of bread; 1/2 bun, bagel, or English muffin
1 ounce of dry ready-to-eat cereal
1/2 cup of cooked cereal, rice, or pasta

Milk Products
1 cup of milk or yogurt
1 1/2 ounces of cheese

Meat, Poultry, Fish, Dry Beans, and Eggs
Daily total about 6 ounces
3 ounces of meat = about the size of a deck of cards
1/2 cup of cooked dry beans/peas = 1 ounce

Adapted from: *Nutrition and Your Health: Dietary Guidelines for Americans*, 3rd ed. U.S. Department of Agriculture, U.S. Department of Health and Human Services, 1990.

WEIGHT CONTROL INFORMATION

Overfat vs. Overweight

Imagine the look of confusion you would get if you walked up to the counter at a delicatessen and asked for 10 pounds. The clerk would probably look annoyed and ask, "10 pounds of what? ham? salami? Swiss cheese?" Yet every day, people say they are going to lose 10 pounds, and no one thinks to ask the same critical question: 10 pounds of what? Would a person claiming to be 10 pounds overweight be satisfied if she or he lost 10 pounds of muscle? Probably not. It would be helpful, then, to differentiate between being overweight and being overfat. To see if you are **overweight**, you can step on a scale, get your weight in pounds (or kilograms), and then consult a height/weight chart. One kilogram is equal to 2.2 pounds. This chart will tell you how many pounds you should weigh for your particular height. Unfortunately, it can't tell you how many of those pounds are fat, muscle, water, or other components of your body. The chart cannot distinguish between a round, soft person and a lean, muscular person as long as they are the same height, weight, and frame size.

Because muscle weighs more than fat, a well-muscled individual weighs more than an average person of the same height. It may surprise you to learn that athletes and other individuals who have low percentages of body fat and well-developed muscles are often classified as overweight according to height/weight charts.

The key is not to find out if you are overweight but rather to find out if you are **overfat**. The body's weight can be broken into two components: fat weight (FW) and lean body mass (LBM). Fat weight is made up of two kinds of fat: subcutaneous fat, which is stored between the skin and the muscles, and intramuscular fat, which is stored between muscle fibers. By pinching yourself you can feel the subcutaneous fat. To picture intramuscular fat, think of how a good, juicy piece of steak, which is a slice of a cow's muscle, is marbled with fat. Lean body mass is derived from the weight of the skeleton, muscles, water, organs, and connective tissue. It is possible to estimate how much of your body is fat weight and how much is lean body mass. This is called assessing your body composition.

Body Composition

Body composition is the relationship between lean body mass and fat weight. It is usually measured and discussed as the percentage of weight that is fat weight. Guidelines for healthy percentages of fat for both men and women are shown in Table 11.2. Note that healthy women have higher levels of fat than healthy men do.

Using the New Food Label

The new food label carries an easier to use nutrition information guide. It is to be required on almost all packaged foods (compared to about 60 percent of products until now). The label below is only an example.

Serving sizes are now more consistent across product lines, are stated in both household and metric measures, and reflect the amounts people actually eat (based on consumer surveys).

The **list of nutrients** covers those most important to the health of consumers, most of whom need to worry about getting *too much* of certain items (fat or sodium, for example), rather than too few vitamins or minerals, as in the past. The numbers next to the nutrients show how much of the nutrient each serving contains.

The label of larger packages must now tell the number of calories per gram of the energy-producing nutrients: fat, carbohydrate, and protein.

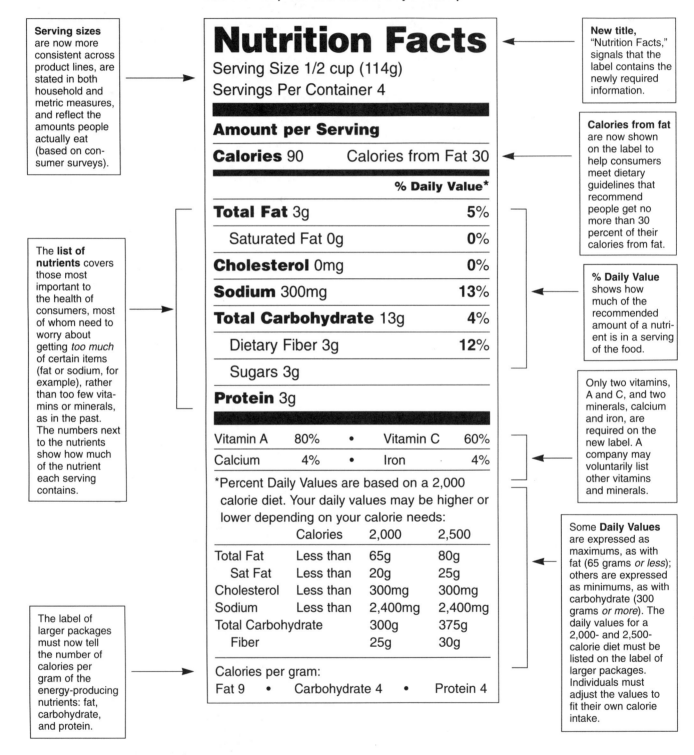

New title, "Nutrition Facts," signals that the label contains the newly required information.

Calories from fat are now shown on the label to help consumers meet dietary guidelines that recommend people get no more than 30 percent of their calories from fat.

% Daily Value shows how much of the recommended amount of a nutrient is in a serving of the food.

Only two vitamins, A and C, and two minerals, calcium and iron, are required on the new label. A company may voluntarily list other vitamins and minerals.

Some **Daily Values** are expressed as maximums, as with fat (65 grams *or less*); others are expressed as minimums, as with carbohydrate (300 grams *or more*). The daily values for a 2,000- and 2,500-calorie diet must be listed on the label of larger packages. Individuals must adjust the values to fit their own calorie intake.

The label content:

Nutrition Facts

Serving Size 1/2 cup (114g)
Servings Per Container 4

Amount per Serving

Calories 90   Calories from Fat 30

% Daily Value*

Total Fat 3g	5%
Saturated Fat 0g	0%
Cholesterol 0mg	0%
Sodium 300mg	13%
Total Carbohydrate 13g	4%
Dietary Fiber 3g	12%
Sugars 3g	
Protein 3g	

Vitamin A	80%	Vitamin C	60%
Calcium	4%	Iron	4%

*Percent Daily Values are based on a 2,000 calorie diet. Your daily values may be higher or lower depending on your calorie needs:

	Calories	2,000	2,500
Total Fat	Less than	65g	80g
Sat Fat	Less than	20g	25g
Cholesterol	Less than	300mg	300mg
Sodium	Less than	2,400mg	2,400mg
Total Carbohydrate		300g	375g
Fiber		25g	30g

Calories per gram:
Fat 9 • Carbohydrate 4 • Protein 4

Source: Food and Drug Administration, 1993.

TABLE 11.2
Body composition: percent fat ratings.

Rating	Women	Men
Very Lean	15 or less	10 or less
Lean	16–17	11–14
Fair	18–25	15–18
Fat	26–29	19–24
Obese	30 or more	25 or more

To illustrate the importance of examining body composition, consider the following two women. Both are 5'4" and 120 pounds and have a small frame size. Both would be considered to be at an ideal weight according to a height/weight chart.

	Person A		*Person B*	
Total weight:	120 lbs.	Total weight:	120 lbs.
Fat weight:	24 lbs.	Fat weight:	36 lbs.
LBM weight:	96 lbs.	LBM weight:	84 lbs.
Percent fat:	20%	Percent fat:	30%
Rating:	**excellent**	Rating:	**poor**

Until groups such as the military, commercial airlines, and cheerleaders realized the difference between overweight and overfat, they were denying valuable, highly fit individuals entry to their programs. Unfortunately, some programs still expect individuals to be at certain weight levels to participate. When a trim, toned individual goes on a crash diet to reach this level, it usually means losing water and muscle to do so. Not only is this highly undesirable, it is also dangerous. People should not be expected to reduce weight levels, they should be expected to attain good body compositions.

There are four common ways to assess body composition. The most accurate is **hydrostatic** or **underwater weighing.** With this method, a person sits on a platform that is attached to a scale. The platform is lowered into the water until the person is totally submerged. After the person exhales as much air as possible, a weight measurement is taken. Since fat floats, a fatter person will weigh less under water than a lean person. The underwater weight is adjusted to account for any air left in the lungs after full exhalation and any gas trapped in the gastrointestinal tract. Finally, an estimate of fat is computed.

This process is fairly costly in both time and facilities. It requires expensive equipment and well-trained technicians. Although you do not have to be a swimmer to participate, this procedure does not work well with individuals who are uncomfortable underwater. If you are comfortable in water and wish to be underwater weighed, check with the physical education department at a uni-

versity or college or with a local sports medicine center. Most places charge a fee for this service. Sometimes when students are learning the procedure, volunteers are needed, in which case you may get it done for free. Be prepared for the process to take at least an hour.

A less expensive, quicker, and more convenient method of assessing body fat is the **skin-fold technique.** It is a little less accurate than underwater weighing, but it still provides a good useful estimate. A caliper is used to measure the thickness of the subcutaneous fat at several sites. The technician uses one hand to pull the skin and subcutaneous fat away from the muscle with his or her thumb and forefinger. With the other hand, she or he uses the caliper to measure the width of the pinched fat (Figure 11.2). The measurements from the different sites are added, and this sum is put into a formula. Some formulas use only one site, some three, and some six or more. Scientists use the multiple-site formulas for accuracy and then recommend the most predictive sites for general use. Some of the most commonly used sites are the back of the arm, just above the hip, the abdomen, just below the shoulder blade, and the front of the thigh. It is easier to train technicians to measure skin folds than to perform underwater weighing. In addition, skin-fold equipment is easily brought to the exercise site. When a fee is charged for this service, it is usually quite small and the test takes only a few minutes.

A third, relatively new, method of analyzing body composition uses what is called a body analyzer or impedance machine. This machine sends a small, harmless electrical impulse through the body. The computer records both the time the impulse takes to travel through

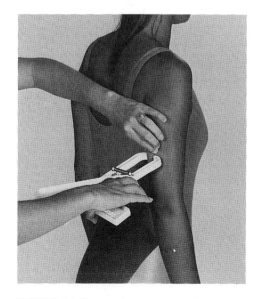

FIGURE 11.2

the body and the amount of resistance the impulse encounters. The impulse travels quickly and with little resistance through water, which makes up a good portion of muscle. It meets more resistance and travels more slowly through fat, since fat is a poor electrical conductor. The computer uses this data to compute your percent body fat. Because this method depends on total body water values, it is important to be at an appropriate level of hydration each time you are tested. Working out before the test or retaining water due to menstruation can throw off the accuracy of this test. Some universities, hospitals, and health clubs have these machines available but usually charge a fee for their service. The test takes only 10 to 15 minutes and is often accompanied by a computer printout that includes your percent fat, recommended weight, and how to attain your recommended weight. Some professionals still question the accuracy of this test, while others believe it to be as accurate as the skin-fold technique when subsequent tests are performed at a similar hydration level.

A fourth fairly accurate measure of body composition can be calculated from girth measurements.

Healthy Weight

For years people have been counseled on how to attain their ideal weight. Now, in an effort to emphasize the importance of body composition (percent fat), the new phrase is "healthy weight." How healthy your weight is depends on how much of it is fat, where on your body it is located, and whether you have weight-related medical problems. Recent research suggests that older people can carry more weight without increased health risks but that excess fat stored in the abdomen (at any age) carries a higher health risk than that in the hips or thighs.

Three methods for calculating your healthy/ideal weight follow. The second two methods retain their use of the phrase "ideal weight" because they were developed using that terminology.

1. Identify your healthy weight by using a height/weight chart. Use Table 11.3 to locate your suggested weight based on height and age.

2. Dr. Kenneth Cooper, in his book *The Aerobics for Total Well-Being,* presents a variation of the Mahoney formula for calculating ideal body weights. Cooper recommends use of this formula when direct measurements of body composition (percent fat) are not available. The ideal weight calculated is intended to represent a weight that includes 15 to 19 percent body fat for men and 18 to 22 percent body fat for women. These calculations are based on average, medium-boned men and women. If you are large boned you need to add 10 percent to the final figure. Women are considered to have large bones if their dominant wrist (wrist supporting the hand they write with) has a circumference larger than 6 1/2 inches. Men are large boned if their dominant wrist measures more than 7 inches.

Women: Height in inches x 3.5 – 108 = ideal weight
Men: Height in inches x 4.0 – 128 = ideal weight

For example, if a man is 6 feet tall and large boned, his ideal weight would be:

72 (6 ft. = 72 in.) x 4.0 – 128 = 160
10% of 160 = 160 x .10 = 16
160 + 16 = 176 lbs. (ideal weight)

3. If you are able to have your percent body fat measured, you can use a third and more accurate method for finding your ideal weight. Subtract your ideal percent fat from your actual percent fat. If the result is a positive number, multiply your present weight by it and subtract the answer from your present weight; if it is a negative number, drop the negative sign, multiply your present weight by it and then add it to your present weight. Here is an example of the calculation for a woman weighing 160 pounds with 26 percent body fat who wants to drop to 20 percent body fat. (Remember to convert the percentage to decimal form before multiplying. For example, 6 percent = 6/100 = 0.06.)

26% – 20% = 6% = 0.06
160 lbs. x 0.06 = 9.6 rounded up to 10
160 – 10 = 150 lbs. (ideal weight)

Try calculating your healthy/ideal weight all three ways, and see how they compare. See Worksheet 8 in the Appendix. If you note a significant discrepancy and you have been able to use the third method, use that figure since percent body fat is directly incorporated in the calculation.

TABLE 11.3
Suggested weights for adults.

| HEIGHT[1] | WEIGHT IN POUNDS[2,3] | |
	19 to 34 years	35 years and over
5'0"	97–128	108–138
5'1"	101–132	111–143
5'2"	104–137	115–148
5'3"	107–141	119–152
5'4"	111–146	122–157
5'5"	114–150	126–162
5'6"	118–155	130–167
5'7"	121–160	134–172
5'8"	125–164	138–178
5'9"	129–169	142–183
5'10"	132–174	146–188
5'11"	136–179	151–194
6'0"	140–184	155–199
6'1"	144–189	159–205
6'2"	148–195	164–210
6'3"	152–200	168–216
6'4"	156–205	173–222
6'5"	160–211	177–228
6'6"	164–215	182–234

[1]Without shoes.

[2]Without clothes.

[3]The higher weights in the ranges generally apply to men, who tend to have more muscles and bone; the lower weights more often apply to women, who have less muscle and bone.

Adapted from: *Nutrition and Your Health: Dietary Guidelines for Americans,* 3rd ed., U.S. Department of Agriculture, U.S. Department of Health and Human Services, 1990.

Weight Adjustment

Three things can happen when you are on a diet: You can gain weight, lose weight, or maintain your weight. As you make changes in an attempt to reach your healthy weight, be sure that you also strive for the ideal balance between fat and lean tissue.

When the number of calories you consume equals the number of calories you expend through physical activity, you are in **energy balance.** Input equals output, and your weight stays the same. When you consume more calories than you expend, you create a positive energy balance, and you gain weight. When you consume fewer calories than you expend, you create a negative energy balance and lose weight. To change your energy balance you can change the number of calories you eat, change the number of calories you burn, or best of all, combine the effects of both.

Weight Loss

Weight loss should be done gradually, just 1/2 to 1 pound a week. This gradual weight loss will keep you off the dieting roller coaster and give you the chance to change your life-style so that the weight stays off. Recent research suggests that yo-yo dieting, that is, alternately gaining and losing weight, may be more hazardous to your health than being overweight. One pound of fat contains 3500 calories; to lose it in one week you have three choices. You can eat 3500 fewer calories per week, which is 500 fewer calories per day; you can eat your same diet and exercise off the 500 calories every day; or you can eat 250 fewer calories and exercise off the other 250. The latter is the easiest approach.

During the first week of a proper diet you may experience a rapid weight loss. After this initial weight loss, work for a steady 1/2 to 1 pound loss per week and don't feel discouraged if your weight remains constant from time to time.

It is a good idea to limit caloric decreases to 500 calories per day or 1000 calories per day if your diet is above 3000 calories. Also, women should be sure to consume a minimum of 1200 calories a day and men a minimum of 1500 calories a day to maintain the basic nutritional needs of the body. Diets that contain fewer calories should be performed only under the care of a physician.

The following is a short list of helpful hints if you are trying to eat fewer calories:

1. Eat planned meals evenly spaced throughout the day to help keep your level of blood sugar steady.

2. Eat fiber-rich foods, which are bulky and will help make you feel full.

3. Eat fresh vegetables and fruits whenever possible. Canned and frozen foods are usually higher in sugar and salt.

4. Chew more slowly so that the meal lasts longer even though you are eating less.

5. Try to eat 75 percent of your calories at breakfast and lunch.

6. Eat low-fat meats whenever possible. Poultry (except duck and goose) and fish are good low-fat choices. Red meat is generally high in fat.

7. Limit the number of times you eat out. This will keep you from eating foods you ordinarily wouldn't cook, and remember, restaurants cook with lots of butter, salt, and fattening sauces.

8. Plan your meals. It's easy to end up eating fat-laden fast foods when you are hungry and there is nothing to eat in the house.

9. Write down everything you eat. Awareness is half the battle.

10. Keep fattening foods out of the house. This helps eliminate temptation.

11. Allow yourself a few sweets during the week, or daily if necessary, so that you aren't tempted to binge on them.

12. Pick one or two areas to improve in at one time. Gradual changes in life-style are easier to accept than radically new ones. In other words, don't try to break two favorite habits at the same time, such as drinking soda and eating chocolate; take them one at a time.

Aerobic exercise five to six times a week, for 30 to 60 minutes per session, at an intensity of about 70 percent of maximal heart rate is recommended for weight loss. If you have not been exercising, you may need to start with fewer days a week, shorter exercise sessions, or both. Consult a fitness professional. People with excess weight may also need to begin with nonweight-bearing activities such as cycling or aquatic exercises. As weight diminishes, weight-bearing activities such as aerobic dance exercise can be added to the program. With a high-frequency program for weight loss (exercise five to six times a week), it would probably be best to limit your participation in aerobic dance exercise to three or four days a week and use a nonweight-bearing or low-impact activity for the other days.

Research evidence indicates that a higher percentage of fat is burned in the lower end of the aerobic target zone. However, this does not necessarily mean that you will burn more fat calories by working at the lower intensity. If you were to exercise at both a low and a moderate intensity for 20 minutes, the total number of calories burned would be greater at the moderate intensity. The more vigorous the exercise, the more calories burned. As exercise intensity goes up, the *percentage* of fat being burned goes down, but the actual number of fat calories burned will increase because the total number of calories burned has increased.

The graphic that follows helps demonstrate this. Imagine that you are eating at a slow pace. You consume 12 food items: 50 percent are carrots, 50 percent are cookies. Eating at a faster pace, you consume 24 items: 33.3 percent are carrots, 33.3 percent are radishes, and

33.3 percent are cookies. Notice that in the first case you ate 6 cookies (50 percent of 12) while in the second case you consumed 8 cookies (33.3 percent of 24). The percentage drops (50 percent to 33.3 percent), but the actual number of cookies increases.

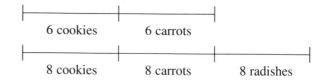

Now turn it around and think of the cookies as fat being burned. Moderate exercise burns more fat calories than low-intensity exercise if the two are performed for the same amount of time. (Note: The percentages used in the cookie/carrot example do not represent the real percentages of fat being burned.)

Increasing the amount of time you exercise at low intensity can offset this difference. Very high intensities burn a lot of calories per minute, but most people find it difficult and uncomfortable to sustain high-intensity exercise. The risk of injury also increases, and mainly carbohydrate is burned.

Fitness professionals recommend that a person expend 300 to 500 calories per exercise session. Individuals at a low fitness level may have to begin with a 200-calorie expenditure, but with gradual overload, they can safely reach a 300-calorie expenditure in about 8 to 12 weeks.

A heavy person will burn more calories than a lighter person doing the same activity since the former must move more weight. Corbin and Lindsey in *Fitness for Life* estimate the following numbers of calories per hour for the body weights listed:

Pounds	Calories/Hour
100	315
120	357
150	420
180	483
200	525

To estimate the number of calories you burn in aerobic dance exercise, perform the following easy calculations:

1. Divide the calories/hour for your weight by 60 to get calories/minute.

2. Multiply the calories/minute by the number of minutes in your class.

A 150-pound person would burn 7 calories per minute (420 ÷ 60). In a 50-minute class this person would burn 350 calories (50 x 7). This class would fulfill the 300- to 500-calorie expenditure requirement for those trying to lose weight.

Besides the obvious calorie-burning effect, exercise also provides other hidden benefits. Your basal metabolic rate is the rate at which your body uses energy to sustain vital functions when you are at rest. When you exercise, your metabolism increases; therefore, you burn more calories. What you may not be aware of is that your metabolic rate remains raised for a period of time following exercise. In addition, every pound of muscle gained through exercise burns an additional 50 calories as compared to a pound of fat. This means you are burning more calories without even trying.

Another hidden benefit of moderate aerobic exercise is the depression of appetite it can cause. Exercising one or two hours before a meal may help you control your appetite. Even vigorous exercise does not stimulate you to eat more calories than you need. What can cause you to overeat is the psychological argument that since you've exercised you can afford to eat more. If you eat preplanned meals you won't fall into that trap.

A final advantage for adding regular exercise to your diet regimen is that fit people start to burn fat more quickly during exercise than unfit people do. It may seem unfair, but fit people have a definite advantage when it comes to weight control. If it is possible, have your percent body fat estimated in about eight-week intervals to see how you are doing. You can also take body measurements to see if you are slimming down. Inches may come off even when pounds don't. Muscle-weight additions may be counteracting fat-weight losses. You can actually lose fat, gain weight, and look better all at the same time!

Weight Maintenance

Maintaining a healthy weight is like standing on your hands. Watch gymnasts carefully, and you will see them make slight adjustments with their fingertips and wrists the whole time they are upside down. Balance is dynamic, not static. To keep your weight and body composition in balance, you constantly need to be aware of your body's needs and activity level and adjust your intake accordingly. The first lesson in this adjustment usually occurs in the late teens when you hear yourself remarking, "I haven't changed my diet at all and suddenly I'm gaining weight." This is probably because you are done growing and don't need as many calories. It may also reflect a

change in lifestyle. Whenever you become more or less physically active, whether the activity is job or exercise related, you need to adjust your diet accordingly. Imagine the different caloric needs of a teenager, a nursing mother, a construction worker, a business executive, and an elderly person. Some of the critical adjustment periods occur during and after pregnancy, around middle age, and at retirement. Listening to your body, adjusting your dietary intake, and maintaining a regular exercise regimen can keep you in balance throughout your life.

Weight Gain

At first it's hard to imagine that anyone would want to gain weight, but there are actually quite a number of people who need weight-gain diets. Certainly undernourished individuals and people recovering from illnesses and accidents fall into this category. On a brighter note, so do athletes and body builders who are trying to put on lean body mass and a few, such as sumo wrestlers, who are actually trying to put on fat as well. Of course, pregnant women must be on weight-gain diets.

To gain lean body weight, you increase your calorie consumption so that it exceeds your calorie expenditure and continue to exercise. If you only increase what you eat and don't exercise, you store the extra calories as fat. (Pregnant women are the exception to this rule.) As mentioned previously, you should add the calories in a way that maintains the recommended percentages of carbohydrates, protein, and fat. A common mistake is to increase protein intake without making a corresponding increase in carbohydrate intake. The body ends up with an excess of protein and too few carbohydrates to fuel the exercise workout.

Muscle (lean body mass) is most effectively increased through progressive resistance exercises such as weight training. Participants in aerobic dance exercise may be able to gain some lean body mass through endurance exercises, depending on their initial strength and whether they use step aerobics, exercise bands, or hand and wrist weights. Aerobic exercise usually reduces fat and maintains lean tissue.

A pregnant woman's weight gain is a little different, but it still involves eating more calories than daily activity expends. The extra calories are used to sustain the higher metabolic rate of the mother and for the growth and development of the baby. Roughly speaking, a pregnant woman needs to consume an extra 300 calories per day. Pregnancy weight gains and exercise programs during and after pregnancy should always be done in consultation with a physician.

Myths and Mistakes

Some of the best nonfiction sellers are diet books. An amazing amount of money is spent on diet books, counseling, and products. Many good diet books and diet plans are available, but a tremendous number also violate the most fundamental rules of good nutrition. They are called fad diets because someone makes a lot of money on them when they first come out, and then they pass into anonymity when dieters find out they don't work. Weight-loss fad diets are easy to spot. They promise quick weight losses and advocate unbalanced diets. They depend on you not caring what kind of weight you lose. When you lose more than 1/2 to 1 pound a week, you will lose beneficial muscle and water weight to do it. For example, you can wrap yourself in plastic and sweat off pounds of water, pop diet pills that cause food to race through your system without being digested, or drink protein drinks and avoid carbohydrates so that you lose substantial amounts of lean tissue and water. If it is fat you are trying to lose, don't get drawn into a fad diet.

Near-starvation diets, crash diets, and prolonged fasting send signals to your body that food is not available and that your life may be threatened. Sensing starvation, the body conserves the energy it has available. In fact, your body may even begin storing the energy as fat to compensate. Your body actually adjusts itself to survive on fewer calories. That's one reason people can survive in near-starvation situations for extended periods of time. Activating this survival instinct makes it more difficult for you to lose fat or, eventually, any form of weight. In fact, many people who are overfat actually eat fewer calories than individuals of normal weight. Once you've been on the crash-diet roller coaster, your body needs some time to readjust to a steady caloric diet.

Unbalanced Diets

Most fad diets stress one type of food. As stated previously, it is important to eat foods from all the food groups to obtain all the essential nutrients. Lack of necessary nutrients can leave you fatigued, depressed, and irritable. Let's take a quick look at what happens when you tip the balance of a diet.

High-protein diets translate into low-carbohydrate and low-fat diets. When your body does not have sufficient quantities of carbohydrates and fats, it uses protein for energy. Nitrogen is a by-product of the protein energy cycle. Too much nitrogen can be toxic. In an effort to clear the body of excess nitrogen, the kidneys combine it with water to make ammonia. The ammonia is excreted in the urine. (It can also be sweated out in small amounts.) When a lot of protein is consumed, the body has to work very hard to clear the nitrogen. Large quantities of water are needed for this process. High-protein diet plans usually tell you to drink an additional 6 to 8 glasses of water per day. Try drinking 16 glasses of water a day; few people can, and so too often the result is dehydration. If the diet is continued, dehydration can become severe, which can lead to kidney failure and death. Even if you don't dehydrate, the low level of carbohydrates will probably make you feel irritable, sick, and fatigued. High-protein diets may also encourage high consumption of meats and dairy foods, which can lead to an unhealthy diet full of saturated fats.

Also watch out for "all you can eat" approaches to dieting. If you eat more calories than you expend, you will gain weight. The origin of the calories doesn't matter; if there are too many they will be stored as fat.

Eating Disorders

Some individuals start to diet and then can't stop. They look in the mirror and continue to see a fat person. One such disease, **anorexia nervosa,** is widespread among women. Men can also suffer from it, but the estimated cases of men with anorexia nervosa are thought to be relatively few at this time. Anorexia nervosa is often associated with life-threatening weight losses and denial of weight loss by the dieter. This disease requires both psychological and medical assistance. If you know anyone suffering from anorexia, do everything possible to get him or her to professional help. Otherwise, your friend may literally starve him or herself to death.

Bulimia, another eating disorder, is characterized by eating regular-sized or large meals and then intentionally emptying the food out of the stomach by self-induced vomiting or the use of laxatives. The lining of the throat and esophagus can become damaged from repeated contact with stomach acids during regurgitation. People suffering from bulimia look healthy, especially since they try to hide their binge-and-purge behavior. Like people who exhibit anorexia, those who suffer from bulimia need immediate psychological and medical attention.

Other Weight Loss Gimmicks

You have already learned how important it is to stay well hydrated. It doesn't make sense, then, to purposely try to lose water. Keeping this in mind, you can avoid some of the diet gimmicks that promise you weight loss and deliver by causing a water-weight loss. For example, rubber suits and plastic wrappings trap in heat so that you sweat out pounds of water. Saunas and whirlpools also sweat out water weight. Some of the diet pills are diuretics that cause you to lose water through frequent urination. Waist and thigh belts temporarily push and sweat water out of targeted areas so that measurements taken immediately after the belt is removed show lost inches. In a couple of hours, the inches are back. Any program that depends on excessive water loss for weight reduction is dangerous and ineffective. You want to lose fat, not water.

Perhaps one of the biggest all-time diet and exercise myths is **spot reducing.** You cannot choose where the fat will come off your body. In general, it will come off gradually all over. If fat tends to accumulate in one place on your body, you can speculate with some certainty that where it went on first, it will come off last. Don't fall into the trap of thinking that because you use your legs to run, you will get rid of the fat on your thighs more quickly. Running on your hands could be just as effective in removing leg fat. Of course, running on your legs will tone up the leg muscles underneath the fat, and running on your hands would certainly help tone your arms.

. . . .

COMMONLY ASKED QUESTIONS

Will exercise increase my appetite?

Easy to moderate exercise actually decreases your appetite. Only with intense exercise does the body (understandably) crave more food. Exercising one to two hours before a meal may help you control your appetite.

Should I eat more when I exercise?

Exercise does burn calories. To maintain your weight you need to take in as many calories as you burn; to lose weight you need to burn more calories than you take in; to gain weight you need to eat more calories than you burn. Depending on what you are trying to accomplish, you may want to increase or decrease your food intake. A woman should consume a minimum of 1200 calories a day, and a man 1500 calories a day unless otherwise advised by a doctor. You should also try to maintain a balance of protein, fat, and carbohydrates. Protein should constitute 10 to 12 percent, carbohydrates 58 to 60 percent, and fat about 30 percent of your diet. A pregnant woman must consume an extra 300 calories a day to support the baby, and if she exercises, she will need to eat more than that.

When should I drink water?

You should stay hydrated at all times. This means that you should drink water about half an hour before class and be sure to replenish your liquids after exercising. Drinking water during class is also a healthy habit. If the class is only an hour long, you probably don't need to stop and get a drink. But if you are thirsty, by all means get one. If you are involved in prolonged exercise, you should drink about half a cup of water every half-hour. It is even more critical to drink water on hot days. Thirst is not a good indicator of your need for water. Drink before you get thirsty.

Will a candy bar before class give me quick energy?

It will give you a short burst of energy and then actually drop your blood sugar. Whenever the blood glucose level gets too high, the liver excretes insulin, which acts to lower the blood sugar. When a lot of sugar is introduced to the system quickly, the liver puts out a lot of insulin. That much insulin ends up dropping the blood sugar below the level it was at prior to the candy. Halfway through class you may suddenly feel very hungry or even sluggish from low blood sugar. You would be better off eating a few crackers before class.

Do I really need to eat breakfast before a morning aerobics class?

Not necessarily. The important thing is that you eat a balanced diet over the course of the day. Many early-morning exercisers eat breakfast after they exercise. However, it would probably be a good idea to hydrate yourself by drinking water or juice before exercising. Other people find they need to eat breakfast to boost their blood sugar before exercising.

Does caffeine improve exercise performance?

Research has shown that caffeine can improve long-distance running performance, but the ingesting of caffeine has two drawbacks. One is that you end up needing to go to the bathroom in the middle of the race. The other is that since caffeine is a diuretic, you will dehydrate more quickly. There doesn't appear to be any advantage in having caffeine before aerobic dance exercise. In fact, in terms of your health, you are better off limiting your caffeine intake, especially if you have high blood pressure.

SUMMARY

Each nutrient plays a special role in your health and well-being, which makes it vital to eat a balanced diet. Being aware of what you are putting in your mouth is the key to eating a balanced, nutritious diet. As an awareness project, record what you eat on a weekday and a weekend day using Worksheets 9A and 9B, then answer the questions on Worksheet 9C. You may be surprised at what you discover.

The bottom line of weight control is that there are no known quick and easy ways to lose fat. You put it on gradually; it must come off gradually. Exercise makes the process a little easier and a lot more fun.

KNOWLEDGE TIPS

1. 58 to 60 percent of the diet should consist of carbohydrates (48 percent complex and natural sugars and 10 percent refined and processed sugars), 10 to 12 percent protein, and not more than 30 percent fat (10 percent saturated, 10 percent monosaturated, and 10 percent polyunsaturated).

2. Carbohydrate is the primary source of energy for the body. Fat is used for energy when prolonged periods of activity demand it. Protein is used for energy only when there is a shortage of available carbohydrate and fat.

3. A balanced diet should depend primarily on foods from the base of the food pyramid: fruits, vegetables, and breads, cereals, rice, and pasta, and secondarily on foods from nearer the top of the pyramid such as milk, yogurt, and cheese, and meats, poultry, fish, dry beans, eggs, and nuts.

4. Vitamins play an essential role in the release of energy from foods.

5. Minerals are inorganic compounds that supply strength and rigidity to body structures and play an important role in the regulation of body processes.

6. Proper hydration is critical to physical health and performance.

7. Plain, cool water is absorbed into the body more quickly than sport drinks or soft drinks.

8. Healthy body composition is characterized by a relatively low percentage of body fat and a relatively high percentage of lean body mass. Healthy women require a higher percentage of fat than do healthy men.

9. During energy balance, caloric intake is equal to caloric expenditure. Weight is gained when intake surpasses expenditure. Weight is lost when expenditure surpasses intake.

10. High-intensity activity burns more calories per minute than low-intensity activity. Yet most people are more successful using longer durations at lower intensities than shorter durations at higher intensities to burn the same number of calories.

11. High-intensity work primarily burns carbohydrate. Moderate-intensity work burns carbohydrate and fat.

12. Aerobic exercise five to six times a week, for 30 to 60 minutes, at a low to moderate intensity is recommended for weight loss.

13. Unbalanced, yo-yo, and rapid weight-loss diets can be dangerous, even life threatening.

14. Anorexia nervosa and bulimia are eating disorders that require immediate medical and psychological attention.

CHAPTER 12

Care and Prevention of Injuries

Pain to gain . . . you'll wind up lame!
No pain, gradual gain . . . win the health fitness game.

If you are in pursuit of health and fitness, there is no reason to beat your body into the ground. Leave the pain and agony to the professionals who are paid handsomely to put their bodies at risk. Some soreness at the beginning of a program is normal, but if you are hurt, exhausted, and run-down after a workout, something is wrong. You should feel temporarily tired and then actually get a lift of energy from the workout.

Aerobic dance exercise is a safe, fun way to exercise, yet injuries do occur. Some injuries are avoidable; others are accidents that can't be prevented. Most of the injuries that occur in aerobic dance exercise can be prevented.

A quick look at the research on aerobic dance injuries can lead you to the wrong conclusions. About 75 percent of instructors and 45 percent of students reported having injuries; this percentage might make one think that aerobic dance exercise is a high-risk activity. Examining the research more carefully, however, shows that most of the injuries were not debilitating, did not require medical treatment, and did not stop the person from exercising. Instructors most likely report more injuries because they spend more time doing the activity. Instructors are often guilty of exceeding the recommended frequency of three to five times per week, which makes them more susceptible to overuse injuries.

Not surprisingly, over half of the reported injuries were below the knee. The most common injuries were shinsplints and tendinitis. In most cases, these are overuse injuries that can be prevented by altering the frequency, intensity, and duration of activity.

Participants who get hooked on aerobic dance exercise sometimes become overzealous. It is a good idea to take at least one day off a week or participate in a nonweight-bearing aerobic activity such as swimming or bicycling once or twice a week. This relieves some of the stress on the lower legs, which is where most of the injuries occur.

When the cause of injury can be identified, the program or facility can be modified to eliminate or minimize the risk of injury. For example, one major cause of shinsplints in aerobic dance exercise is impact stress. Some of the modifications made to minimize shinsplints have been the production of better-designed aerobic shoes, the installation and use of better floors, and the introduction of low-impact aerobics.

Participants can prevent many injuries by increasing their strength and flexibility. For example, they can often relieve back pain by adopting a good stretching and strengthening program. Good posture and exercise technique are also critical to injury prevention.

People who are beginning a program and those with a history of orthopedic problems run a slightly higher risk of injury. To reduce this elevated risk, simply start slowly, overload gradually, and avoid exercises that hurt.

Unfortunately, there will always be unforeseeable accidents. When an accident occurs, the best thing to do is to administer prompt, proper first aid. Make sure the facility where you exercise is prepared to handle emergency situations.

Learn how to put prevention in your program. Listed below are some of the injuries that can occur during aerobic dance exercise. The common causes, preventive actions, and proper first aid for each injury are listed.

FOOT INJURIES

Blister

DEFINITION   Inflammation of the skin that results in a collection of fluid below the skin.

SYMPTOMS   Hot and red skin.

CAUSE   Friction of the skin against something else.

PREVENTION   Wear shoes that fit properly; wear socks. Put bandages or skin tape or rub petroleum jelly over the heel and other high-risk locations before breaking in new shoes or doing a long day of aerobics.

TREATMENT   Apply ice, rest, and put a felt or moleskin donut around the blister so that no further rubbing will occur. If the blister opens, wash with soap and water, dry, apply antibiotic ointment, and cover the area. Do not intentionally pop a blister. If it is in a very uncomfortable location and must be drained, use a sterilized needle to make a small hole in the lower side, drain, use antibiotic ointment, and cover. Do not remove the skin.

Bunion

DEFINITION   Bump that forms on the side of the big or little toe. Toe may turn inward.

SYMPTOMS   Burning, tenderness, swelling, redness, pain, and misalignment of toe.

CAUSES   Wearing shoes that are too narrow or too short.

PREVENTION   Wear shoes that fit well.

TREATMENT   Reduce friction with pad or new shoes. Soak in cool water. See a physician.

Metatarsalgia

DEFINITION   Irritation of the nerves that lie between the metatarsal bones. (Metatarsals are the bones between the toes and the arch.)

SYMPTOMS   Pain under the ball of the foot.

CAUSES   Shifting forward of the protective fat pad under the ball of the foot from excessively landing on it; overuse.

PREVENTION   An aerobic shoe with good metatarsal (forefoot) padding, good jump-landing technique, and resilient floor. Avoid overuse.

TREATMENT   Ice, rest, and cushioned foot pads. If the pain persists, see a physician. You may need metatarsal lifts or orthotics.

Plantar Fascitis

DEFINITION   Strain to the broad sheet of connective tissue that runs from the heel to the metatarsals, which supports the longitudinal arch. When weight is shifted to the ball of the foot, the tension held by this connective tissue equals twice the body's weight.

SYMPTOMS   Pain just in front of the heel where the connective tissue connects to the heel bone. May feel bruised. Pain may also radiate along the arch.

CAUSES   A rapid increase in activity that requires pushing off the ball of the foot, particularly on a hard surface; wearing unsupportive shoes.

PREVENTION   Work into a new program gradually. Wear shoes that support the arches. Develop calf flexibility.

TREATMENT   Soak in cool water, buy new shoes or arch supports. If it persists, see a physician; you may need orthotics or anti-inflammatory drugs.

Morton's Neuroma

DEFINITION Localized swelling of the sensory nerve that lies between the metatarsals (bones in the ball of the foot) and innervates the toes.

SYMPTOMS Pain radiating up between the third and fourth toes.

CAUSES Overuse, too much running on the ball of the foot.

PREVENTION Well-cushioned aerobic shoes. Avoid overuse with a practical program. Use a metatarsal arch pad (a felt pad that fits under the ball of the foot).

TREATMENT See a physician.

SHIN INJURIES

Shinsplints

DEFINITION This is a general term for pain on the front or side of the lower leg. Some believe the pain comes from minute tearing of the muscle sheath from the shin bone membrane. Others believe the pain comes from damage caused by excessive vibration of the bone.

SYMPTOMS Pain and aching in the shin area after and sometimes during exercise. May be specific areas of tenderness or swelling over the bone.

CAUSES Impact stress from a hard floor, poorly cushioned shoes, too much jumping, poor foot mechanics, poor posture, fallen arches, insufficient warm-up, fatigue, training too fast or too soon, poor exercise technique.

PREVENTION Dance on a resilient floor with good arch-supporting shoes and proper footwork. Strengthen the foot muscles and muscles that surround the shin, especially the anterior tibialis. Stretch calves well before working out. Also keep shins warm before and during class. Warm-up socks are helpful for this.

TREATMENT Ice shins for 20 to 30 minutes following exercise. You may want to freeze water in a paper cup and use it to massage your shins. Just peel down the cup as the ice melts.

If any bruising, swelling, or specific point tenderness occurs, stop exercising and rest your legs. If pain persists or worsens, consult a physician. You may need to take an anti-inflammatory drug or be fitted for orthotics.

Some individuals get relief from having their arches, shins, or both taped—consult an athletic trainer or podiatrist. Some people also get relief by running backward.

If your shins start to bother you during a class, try modifying the movements to a low-impact style. If you are at a health club, you can leave the floor during the standing aerobics to bicycle, row, or do stairs, and then rejoin the class for body toning exercises.

Stress Fracture

DEFINITION Very thin, undisplaced hairline break in a bone.

SYMPTOMS Pain along the lower leg bones. If it is a stress fracture in the lower leg, it will hurt before, during, and after class and even when you get off your feet. Painful when you touch it, especially in one area.

CAUSES Same as shinsplints.

PREVENTION Wear cushioned, supportive shoes, avoid overuse and nonresilient surfaces.

TREATMENT See a physician. Stress fractures are difficult to diagnose because they don't show up on X-rays until calcium deposits are made during the healing process. Once diagnosed, the fractured part of the leg may be immobilized in a cast.

KNEE INJURIES

Chondromalacia Patella

DEFINITION Roughening or softening of the joint surface of the knee cap (patella).

SYMPTOMS Pain when patella is pressed on, maybe creaking and popping noises. May hurt when climbing stairs or kneeling. Knee pain while exercising.

CAUSES Knee cap may be sliding out of alignment and causing irritation. Cartilage may be inflamed or degenerating. May be caused by deep knee bends or other exercises that stress the knee.

PREVENTION Perform a good warm-up. Avoid deep knee bends and knee hyperextension positions. Strengthen the muscles that surround and support the knee, using straight-leg exercise. Stretch legs, especially the hamstrings and calves.

TREATMENT Ice the knee. See a physician. Strengthen supporting muscles.

Meniscal Injuries

DEFINITION   Strains or tears of the cartilage that stabilizes the knee joint.

SYMPTOMS   Acute pain, popping noise, swelling, knee may "give out" or lock.

CAUSES   Rotation or twisting of the knee joint beyond normal limitations. Foot remaining planted when the body turns so that the knee is forced to accept the rotational force. A floor with too much cushion allows the foot to sink into it and remain planted. Sticky floors or treaded shoes on nonslip surfaces may also cause the foot to remain planted. Injury can also be caused by working the knee joint with too much weight.

PREVENTION   Select the appropriate shoe for the surface. Select the best possible surface. Use workout routines that don't require sudden pivots or turns, particularly on soft floors. Work with reasonable amounts of weight during leg exercises. Overload gradually and strengthen the supporting muscles.

TREATMENT   Support the back of the knee and pack the knee in ice. Move the person only if the knee is supported. Keep injured person warm and call a doctor. Joint may have to be aspirated (excess fluid removed from the joint).

. . . .

MULTIPLE SITE INJURIES

Strain

DEFINITION   Injury to a muscle or a tendon. (**Tendons** connect muscles to bone; e.g., the Achilles tendon connects the calf muscle to the heel.)

SYMPTOMS   There are three degrees of injury. First-degree symptoms: local pain and tenderness usually accompanied by swelling and pain. Exercise may be continued when pain and swelling are absent and range of motion is complete. Second-degree symptoms: pain with muscle movement, muscle spasm, increased swelling, and tearing of tissue. Do not continue exercise. Third-degree symptoms: severe pain and disability, severe muscle spasms, and complete tearing of tissue. Do not continue exercise.

CAUSES   Pushing a muscle or tendon beyond its normal range, often by a ballistic movement before the body is fully warmed up. May also occur from overuse or flinging the arms, especially when arm weights are used. Older persons are more prone to injury.

PREVENTION   Warm up and stretch well before working out. Strengthen both agonists and antagonists.

TREATMENT   Rest, ice, compress, and elevate (RICE) the injured muscle or tendon. If pain is acute or persists, see a physician. Do not move anyone who has a third-degree strain. Call a doctor; surgery may be necessary.

Sprain

DEFINITION   Injury to a ligament. (**Ligaments** attach bones to bones.)

SYMPTOMS   First-degree symptoms: twinge of discomfort, slight skin discoloration from internal bleeding, some ligament fiber damage. Exercise may be continued when pain and swelling are absent and range of motion is complete. Second-degree symptoms: pain, swelling, loss of function for several minutes, tender to the touch, loss of strength, definite tear of fibers. Do not continue exercise. Third-degree symptoms: severe pain and swelling, discoloration of skin, complete tear of the ligament, loss of function. Do not continue exercise.

CAUSES   Any movement that pulls two connected bones apart more than a normal amount.

PREVENTION   Warm up and stretch before working out. Exercise regularly so that ligaments are strengthened. Overload gradually and remember that ligament strength gains are usually slower than cardiorespiratory gains. When your heart says keep going, check in with the rest of your body. Strengthen muscles that surround joints so that they can minimize the stress put on the ligaments. Avoid exercises that put pressure on ligaments, and do exercises that strengthen muscles. For example, squats and lunges strengthen the legs as long as you don't bend the knee too much; deep knee bends stress the ligaments, and because the muscles are in a weak mechanical position, they can't help the ligaments.

TREATMENT   Rest, ice, compress, and elevate (RICE) the injured part. If pain is acute or persists, consult a physician. If it is a third-degree sprain, do not move the person. Keep the person warm and call a doctor. Surgical repair may be necessary.

Tendinitis

DEFINITION   Chronic inflammation or irritation of a tendon. Microscopic tears in the tendon tissue may be the cause of the inflammation.) In aerobics, the most commonly injured tendons are the Achilles, shoulder, and elbow.

SYMPTOMS   Area may be painful to the touch, warm and swollen. Skin may be red.

CAUSES   Repeated excessive stretching of a tendon, excessive running or jumping especially on hard surfaces, flinging of arms particularly when wrist weights are used.

PREVENTION   Use careful, deliberate movements rather than flinging movements. Gradually overload. Warm up and stretch out prior to vigorous activity.

TREATMENT   Ice and rest the tendon. If pain is acute, see a physician. May require anti-inflammatory drugs or surgery.

Bursitis

DEFINITION   Inflammation or irritation of a bursa. Bursas are fluid-filled sacks found around the body at sites where friction might occur, such as where muscle tendons and sheaths cross over bones.

SYMPTOMS   Localized inflammation, pain, swelling, and heat.

CAUSES   Overstretching of the Achilles tendon, direct blow to the elbow or knee, pressure on an area such as the knee, or overuse of a joint, such as the deltoid at the shoulder through unaccustomed overhead arm activity.

PREVENTION   Avoid overuse of muscles and joints. Avoid kneeling on a hard floor. Use gradual overloads, especially when adding resistance through weights or exercise bands. Use good exercise technique.

TREATMENT   Ice and compress the area. If pain or loss of motion persists, consult a physician.

Muscle Cramp

DEFINITION   Painful muscle contraction that will not voluntarily release.

SYMPTOMS   Acute pain.

CAUSES   Fatigue or heat induced. (Also common among pregnant women, possibly due to chemical changes.)

PREVENTION   Warm up and stretch before vigorous exercise. Stretch a muscle following a strength work-out. Stretch whenever slight muscle cramping occurs. Cool the calves in very hot weather by removing warm-up socks and wearing lightweight tights or shorts. Hydrate with water prior to exercise and if cramps develop.

TREATMENT   Stretch and massage the muscle. (You can also ice the opposing muscle because its contraction will cause the other muscle to stretch.)

HEAT-RELATED INJURIES

Heat Cramp

See Muscle Cramp.

Heat Exhaustion

DEFINITION   Overheating of the body.

SYMPTOMS   Muscle spasms or cramping, cold clammy skin, chills, nausea, dizziness, and profuse sweating.

CAUSES   Inability to dissipate heat because the room is too hot or humid for the level of activity. Sometimes aerobic studios are not properly ventilated or the cooling systems are insufficient. Situations can also arise when the exercise room shares air from a pool.

PREVENTION   Exercise in a well-ventilated, controlled-temperature environment. Adjust the exercise level so that it is safe for the environment. Keep yourself well hydrated.

TREATMENT   Drink water and cool the body by going to a cooler place or using ice. Rest.

Heat Stroke

DEFINITION   Inability of the body to handle heat stress. This is a medical emergency. The core temperature is rising, and brain damage and death can result.

SYMPTOMS   Dry hot skin, pale or flushed skin, nausea, dizziness, faintness, weakness, or exhaustion. Skin may be hot and dry or still sweating if exercise has just stopped.

CAUSES   Overexposure to a hot or hot and humid environment.

PREVENTION   Keep yourself well hydrated. Do not exercise in very hot weather or when the heat and humidity combine to cause a hazardous condition. Although these conditions do not occur often in most places, a wise participant will not continue to take a class if the air conditioner fails or if he or she is attending a class outdoors on a very hot day. Such a day may be good for aqua aerobics.

TREATMENT   Immediately cool the body. Put person in a cold shower or dump cold water all over him or her. Call an ambulance immediately.

. . . .

OTHER HEALTH CONCERNS

Exercising While Pregnant

Exercise is a positive health habit that in most cases can be continued through pregnancy. It is important, however, to recognize the new demands on your body and adjust accordingly. A pregnant woman who plans to continue or begin an exercise program during pregnancy should consult with her physician first. It is better to start an exercise program before pregnancy, but it is possible to begin light exercising during pregnancy. A special beginners' program for pregnant women may be the best way to get started. Women who have been exercising regularly prior to conception may be able to continue in a regular class for a while, as long as they make appropriate adjustments to their level of intensity. As pregnancy advances many women prefer special classes or turn to nonweight-bearing activities such as cycling.

The American College of Obstetricians and Gynecologists (ACOG) developed a set of guidelines for exercise. These guidelines are understandably conservative and were developed with the formerly inactive woman in mind. ACOG recommends that a pregnant woman stay below a heart rate of 140 beats per minute, limit vigorous exercise to 15 minutes, and after the fourth month, avoid exercises that require her to lie on her back. Complications in a pregnancy may require cessation of all exercise. For more information contact your local hospital, physician, or ACOG.

If your doctor agrees that exercise is healthy for you, discuss frequency, intensity, and time with him or her. Be aware that during pregnancy your ligaments will be looser and more relaxed than normal, so you must take care not to overstretch. As you put on weight, you will also experience a changing balance point. You may periodically feel clumsy or uncoordinated, but try not to let it frustrate you. You can always simplify steps or walk in place and enjoy the music. Finally, make sure your instructor is aware of your pregnancy and provide your instructor with the phone numbers of your physician, the hospital, and the relative you want contacted in case of an emergency. After giving birth, don't start exercising until you have your physician's clearance, and then do not stress your body too much. With the right precautions, exercise can enhance your pregnancy and help you regain your shape after giving birth.

Diabetes and Exercise

If you have diabetes and are planning to begin an exercise program, discuss it with your physician. If you take insulin shots, make sure you know when and where to inject them. For example, if you inject into a leg muscle just before class, the muscle activity during class will cause the insulin to circulate through your body much more rapidly than normal. Participants with diabetes should also avoid taking a class on an empty stomach. Prevent sudden low blood sugar by eating something like crackers and juice about half an hour before class. It is also a good idea to pack fruit or some other snack in your gym bag in case complications arise. Foot care is also important. Wear good socks and keep your feet dry and free of athlete's foot. If you experience foot problems, see your physician immediately. In addition to providing the usual benefits, regular moderate exercise can help a person with diabetes maintain normal blood glucose levels and in some cases may reduce the need for insulin. Any changes should, of course, be made under the guidance of a physician.

Asthma and Exercise

Some people experience exercise-induced asthma. The labored breathing caused by bronchial constriction may discourage people with asthma from exercising. But research has shown that increased aerobic fitness raises the exertion level at which symptoms begin to occur. Therefore, people with asthma can and should exercise. If you do experience exercise-induced asthma, try to recognize early symptoms and then lower your intensity or take a break if necessary. You should also bring your bronchodilator medication to class in case of severe symptoms. Long, gradual warm-ups also seem to ease symptoms. Be sure to consult with your physician and then let your instructor know that you have asthma. Work together to set an appropriate level of intensity and work on increasing symptom-free time.

Back Care and Exercise

An alarmingly high number of people experience lower back pain some time in their lives. Strong flexible muscles, good posture, and good exercise technique can all help prevent lower back pain. Tips throughout this book explain how to take care of your back, but I would like to summarize some of those thoughts and introduce one last exercise. An additional set of guidelines for back care appears in the Appendix. Rules to remember:

· Stand with your knees slightly flexed.

· Keep your pelvis straight, allowing a normal (not exaggerated) curvature of the spine.

· Stabilize your back during exercises by contracting your abdominal muscles.

· Avoid back-arching or standing flat-back positions.

· Strengthen your abdominal and back muscles.

· Develop good flexibility in both the hamstrings and the hip flexors (quadriceps and iliopsoas).

· Use your legs when lifting heavy objects.

· Turn with your feet, not your waist, when putting down heavy objects.

· Carry heavy objects close to your body.

· And finally, one last exercise you can perform anywhere, anytime—and should! Tuck your chin in and pull your shoulders back slightly. You will feel immediate relief in your upper back and neck.

COMMONLY ASKED QUESTIONS

Should I exercise when I'm sick?

No, exercise is a stressor. When your body is trying to fight off infection, it needs rest, not stress.

How can I tell if I am overtraining?

One way to tell is to monitor your resting heart rate first thing in the morning. If it starts to increase, give yourself a day off. Another sign of overtraining is loss of strength. Strength gains are made only when the muscle has enough time to rebuild between exercise bouts. Chronic injury, lethargy, lack of motivation, and chronic fatigue are all signs of overuse.

Why do I get muscle cramps during class?

Most cramps occur when a muscle is fatigued. If you experience cramping, stretch out better before class, lower your exercise intensity, and stretch the muscle more often during class. Sometimes poor choreography overworks one set of muscles. This can make you stiff and sore or make you cramp. The best choreography works both muscles in a muscle pair. If you know that you worked one muscle harder than another, do a set of exercises to balance the workout.

Other causes for cramping included overheated muscles, dehydration, and electrolyte imbalance. Drinking water prevents heat cramps. Taking salt pills to prevent heat cramps is not a good idea. The salt can upset your stomach during exercise, and furthermore, most American diets contain more salt than is recommended. Only in rare cases is a salt supplement required. Some people find that eating a banana (a good source of potassium) helps prevent cramping. A complex vitamin B supplement may also help chronic cramping. Consult your physician if cramping is persistent.

Am I working hard enough if I don't sweat much?

Sweat is not a good measure of exercise intensity. Different people sweat different amounts and in different places. Some sweat profusely before they even cross the training threshold. Others hardly sweat at all. Heart rate is a better indicator of intensity.

Men usually sweat more than women because they have more sweat glands and more muscle. When muscle is working, heat is generated—the more muscle the more heat. Sweat is a good thing. The evaporation of sweat cools the body.

Sometimes I feel dizzy during class. Can I prevent that?

Dizziness can be caused by a number of things. It may be brought on by low blood sugar. This is often the case when people take a morning class without eating anything for breakfast. Another cause can be heat stress. Wear loose, comfortable clothing and drink water.

Dizziness may also be a sign of illness. If dizziness occurs, stop exercising and walk around. If you feel as though you are going to faint, lie down and elevate your feet. If dizziness persists, check with a doctor.

Is it good to "go for the burn"?

The burn is the feeling you get when your muscles are working so hard that oxygen cannot be supplied to them fast enough to produce energy. This ischemia (lack of oxygen) and the accumulation of lactic acid make your muscles feel heavy and sometimes cause a burning sensation. If you are trying to work aerobically, the burn is counterproductive because it is a product of heavy anaerobic exercise. Body toning exercises are anaerobic, and it is during these exercises that you are most likely to feel the burn. If you do, you should change the exercise or take a short break to allow blood to circulate through the limb. This will enable you to exercise longer and eventually develop better endurance.

Will curl-ups flatten my tummy?

Curl-ups will tone the abdominal muscles, but only aerobic exercise removes fat from the body. A combination of aerobic and body toning exercises will result in a trim, toned midsection.

I prefer to do my muscle endurance exercises at a fast pace. Is this okay?

No. When you move a limb quickly in one direction and then quickly back the other way, you strengthen only the turnaround points. The muscles work hard at these two points to stop the fast-moving limb and get it going the other way. Unfortunately, little strengthening occurs during the rest of the range of motion because momentum carries the weight of the limb. If you want strong muscles throughout a range of motion, exercise at a moderate pace so that momentum is eliminated. Moderately paced movements also prevent injury.

Sometimes I get bored with aerobic dance exercise. Is that normal?

Yes; everyone can experience burnout. You can take a break from aerobic dancing by getting involved with another kind of aerobic exercise. The important thing is to continue exercising!

What is cross training, and should I do it?

To cross train is to use two or more types of exercises to train. For example, you can train aerobically using both swimming and aerobic dance exercise. Because each activity uses your muscles differently, you will get a more complete workout. But you do not need to cross train to achieve health-related fitness—each activity by itself provides a good aerobic workout. Cross training can help combat boredom and prevent overuse injury, two reasons that people drop out of programs. Cross train if it appeals to you and if you want to increase your skill and ability in more than one activity.

I get a side ache (stitch) when I exercise. Why does this happen, and what should I do?

A side ache is usually caused by a bubble of gas caught in your system. Eating too close to the time of exercise or starting your exercise too quickly may cause it. To relieve a side ache, try stretching up with the arm on the side giving you distress. If it continues, slow down your activity and try doing some side and waist stretches.

Will I make even greater gains if I exercise at an intensity above 80 percent of my HR$_{max}$reserve?

The greatest aerobic fitness gains are obtained between 60 to 80 percent of HR$_{max}$reserve. Working above 80 percent will continue to improve your fitness level but in much smaller increments. And remember, intense anaerobic exercise is difficult to sustain. During anaerobic exercise, carbohydrates become the main source of energy and as a result the burning of fat is reduced. Exercisers also face a higher risk of injury in the high-intensity range. The optimal range for health benefits is 60 to 80 percent of HR$_{max}$reserve or 70 to 85 percent of HRmax.

I don't feel like I'm getting a workout when I exercise in my training heart rate range (THR). Why?

There may be several reasons for this. You may have calculated your training range incorrectly. Check your figures. Or you may not be counting your pulse accurately.

Have someone else take your pulse and compare it to your count. If you have calculated and counted correctly, it might be that the formulas are not working for you. Remember, they are based on the average person. If you have the opportunity, run a treadmill test to find out your true range. You can also try working with the rating of perceived exertion scale (Chapter 3). It is also possible that you are used to competitive levels of training and need time to adjust to the feel of exercise just for the health of it. Discuss your situation with a health fitness professional.

SUMMARY

Many injuries are preventable. Avoid the kinds of exercises that cause injury; you must take responsibility for keeping yourself injury free. If an unforeseen accident does occur, seek proper first aid and then consult a doctor. When you return to class after recovering from an injury, be sure to start out slowly to prevent reinjury.

Much of the fitness information available today is very easy to understand; some of it is very complex; much of it can be misunderstood. Like dieting, exercise information is regularly abused in an attempt to sell quick-fix equipment and programs. The best way to avoid being misinformed is to read exercise literature written by the experts and to ask questions of the experts you have available. Ask your instructors questions—they will welcome the opportunity to enhance your knowledge.

KNOWLEDGE TIPS

1. You can prevent injuries by wearing good shoes, exercising on a resilient surface, using good exercise technique, maintaining proper alignment throughout the class, and modifying exercises to suit your ability.

2. Most of the injuries that occur during aerobic dance exercise are the result of overuse.

3. Only a very small percentage of aerobic dance–exercise injuries require the person to stop exercising.

4. Instructors receive more injuries than students, probably because instructors spend more time doing aerobics and are therefore more susceptible to overuse injuries.

5. The immediate first aid for a sprain or strain is RICE: rest, ice, compression, and elevation.

6. Aerobic dance exercise is one of the safest activities available.

CHAPTER 13

Now That You're Fit...

Health-related physical fitness is a lifetime endeavor. It is relatively easy to exercise in a classroom setting since you are surrounded by other exercisers, recreational facilities, and a teacher. As you leave this course, your surroundings will change; I hope your exercising habits will not. To help you take the first step toward continuing your commitment to a lifetime of aerobic conditioning, this chapter offers a few suggestions on how to find aerobic dance exercise outside this college course.

Exercise programs are offered at a variety of places, including recreation departments, continuing education programs, YMCAs, YWCAs, hospitals, and private clubs. The idea is to find a quality program that fits your needs. Knowing some of the characteristics of good programs can help you formulate questions and make decisions as you look at the possibilities in your area. When you visit a fitness facility, you should receive a full tour and a thorough explanation of the classes that are offered, available equipment, daily hours, and fee structure. When you first join a fitness program you should receive an orientation to the facility and programs. This orientation should include an introduction to the facility and equipment, a medical history, a fitness evaluation, and exercise prescription.

A member of the staff should show you the entire facility and teach you how to use available equipment. A good program will always have someone to help you with exercise questions, equipment, and fitness testing. Sometimes this person is the aerobics instructor, sometimes an additional staff person.

The medical history you complete allows the instructor to work in an informed environment, to decide whether certain exercises should be modified. Find out if the medical questionnaire is used or just filed away.

The fitness evaluation provides baseline data about your personal fitness level. Based on this information, goals and a plan of action can and should be formulated. The program should offer periodic testing to measure improvement, provide motivation, and evaluate the effective-

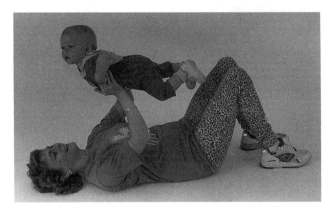

FIGURE 13.1
A lifetime of fitness.

ness of your exercise program. The fitness evaluation should include measures of cardiorespiratory endurance, muscular strength and endurance, body composition, and flexibility. The person conducting these tests should be knowledgeable in fitness testing.

Watch the aerobics class you wish to join from beginning to end. See if it includes a warm-up (core and stretch), 20 to 30 minutes of aerobics, a standing cooldown, body toning exercises (time permitting), and a cool-down stretch. Listen for heart rate or other intensity checks during the class. Check the starting and finishing times for promptness. Make sure you like the instructor's style, and check to see if there is room for you in the class. Check to see if enrollment is limited and if it guarantees you space on the floor. If the class runs on a first come, first served basis, be sure you will have enough time to arrive early.

Program variety allows you to select a class that most closely fits your fitness goals and interests. Many programs now offer a variety of workout levels. Check with the instructor to find out what constitutes a beginning, intermediate, and advanced class. Different programs use different criteria for establishing class levels.

As a guideline, beginning classes usually have a 15- to 20-minute standing aerobics section, work at near-threshold intensities, and do shorter sections of floor work. Intermediate classes work aerobically for a minimum of 20 minutes and include fairly demanding floor exercises. Advanced classes work at high intensities and may include workouts with weights and rubber bands. Their aerobic section may be 20 to 30 minutes long.

Low-impact and step classes are offered in both low and high intensities. Find out when each kind meets and whether weights and exercise bands are used and supplied.

Special classes may be taught for children, elderly persons, pregnant women (pre/postnatal), people with dis-

abilities, and people who are overfat. Each class should use music and techniques appropriate to the people involved. Instructors should be qualified to teach these specialty classes.

Select a program that can meet your needs now and in the future. For instance, if you are very active now and are considering becoming pregnant, select a program that has both an advanced class and a pre/postnatal class. That makes it easy to switch from one to the other at the appropriate time. If you can attend only one time of day and one class, look for an instructor who has experience working with different levels of classes and who is capable of effectively handling people of different fitness levels in one class.

Although major injuries are rare in aerobic dance exercise, it is always comforting to know that the program or facility has an emergency procedure. Check for easy exits, sprinklers, and an available telephone. In addition, the instructors and staff should be educated and certified in cardiopulmonary resuscitation (CPR) and standard first aid. Ice should be readily available in the event of a strain or sprain.

The following is a quick checklist of items to look for as you select an exercise facility. The perfect facility is difficult to find and generally expensive to join, so decide which items are most important to you and look for them.

1. The facility should be in a convenient location near home or work.

2. The building should be well ventilated and the temperature set at a comfortable exercise temperature (about 65 to 70 degrees F).

3. The lighting should be good quality and nonglare.

4. The whole facility, including locker rooms, should be clean and well supplied even at peak hours.

5. The water in pools and whirlpools should appear clear and clean.

6. Mirrors should be strategically placed so that you can check your alignment during exercise.

7. The best aerobics floor is a wooden floor with air space underneath it so that it "gives." Carpet over cement is very hard on shins. Heavy padding can have a tendency to grab your shoe, making changes of direction hazardous.

8. There should be 25 square feet of space available for each person on the aerobics floor. (The absolute minimum is 9 square feet.)

9. The stereo equipment and facility acoustics should project music with a quality sound. The instructor should also be easily heard—many now wear wireless microphones.

10. The aerobics instructor should stand on a platform for easy visibility. Mirrors also enhance visibility for both the instructor and the participant.

Selecting a facility is similar to buying a car. Shop around and visit last the place you think you'll like the most. Many clubs offer a first visit (or initial visit) discount. If you have shopped the competition and like what you see, you'll be able to take advantage of the discount. However, the initial visit discount should not pressure you into buying. Clubs often offer a membership plan on your second visit that is similar to the first plan. Check the life of the club before buying a long-term membership: Small businesses have a high rate of closure. You won't want to purchase a lifetime membership or even a two- to three-year membership if the club is going to go out of business. Some states now have legislation that makes the sale of lifetime memberships illegal.

Many clubs will not disclose their membership costs over the telephone. Most recreation, school, or church groups will tell you the cost of the program, if any, over the telephone.

In all cases, the facility should be well staffed with friendly, qualified people. Some locations include a juice bar, weights, a pool, a sauna, a hairdresser, a nursery, and other amenities. Determine what is important to you before you go to look, so that you won't be distracted by things you don't need and won't use. Find the best facility for you at the most affordable price.

. . . .
SUMMARY

Make finding a place to continue your aerobic dance exercise a priority. In addition to staying fit, going to exercise class is a great way to meet other health-conscious people who look good and feel good just like you!

KNOWLEDGE TIPS

1. Before looking for a fitness facility, make a prioritized list of features to look for.

2. Visit a facility at the same time of day you will be most likely to use it.

3. Look for a fitness facility that will take you on a complete tour, have you complete a medical/health questionnaire, give you a fitness evaluation, explain how to use the equipment, help you get started in an exercise program, and have someone available for consultation on an ongoing basis.

4. Look over the whole facility. Check for cleanliness, ventilation, good lighting, sound acoustics, well-maintained equipment, and a good aerobics floor.

5. Check the instructors' educational backgrounds and ask whether they are certified in CPR, first aid, and aerobic dance exercise.

6. Observe, from start to finish, the aerobics class you wish to join.

7. Consider the financial commitment carefully. Be sure to ask about all the plans.

8. Join and have fun!

Bibliography

Alter, J. *Stretch & Strengthen.* Boston: Houghton Mifflin, 1986.

———. *Surviving Exercise.* Boston: Houghton Mifflin, 1983.

American Alliance for Health, Physical Education, Recreation and Dance. *Health Related Physical Fitness: Test Manual.* Reston, VA: American Alliance for Health, Physical Education, Recreation, and Dance, 1980.

American College of Sports Medicine. *Guidelines for Exercise Testing and Exercise Prescription.* 3rd ed. Philadelphia: Lea and Febiger, 1986.

———. "Position Statement: Proper and Improper Weight Loss Programs." *Medicine and Science in Sports and Exercise* 15 (No. 1, 1983): ix–xiii.

———. "The Recommended Quantity and Quality of Exercise for Developing and Maintaining Cardiorespiratory and Muscle Fitness in Healthy Adults." *Medicine and Science in Sports and Exercise* 22 (No. 2, 1990): 265–74.

American Dietetic Association. "Position Statement on Nutrition and Physical Fitness." *Journal of the American Dietetic Association* 76 (1980): 437–43.

Anshel, M. H. *Aerobics for Fitness.* Edina, MN: Bellwether Press, 1985.

Arnheim, D. *Modern Principles of Athletic Training.* 6th ed. St. Louis, MO: Times Mirror/Mosby, 1985.

Astrand, P. O., and K. Rodahl. *Textbook of Work Physiology.* 2nd ed. New York: McGraw-Hill, 1977.

Barnard, R. J. "The Heart Needs a Warm-Up Time." *The Physician and Sportsmedicine* 4 (No. 1. 1976): 40.

Belt, C. R. "Injuries Associated with Aerobic Dance." *American Family Physician* 41 (June 1990): 1769–72.

Bishop, J. G., and D. Booth. "Injury Prevention and Care of Aerobic Dance-Exercise Injuries." *National Aerobics Training Association Manual.* Mesa, AZ: National Aerobics Training Association, 1986.

Blair, S. N. "Physical Activity, Physical Fitness, and Health." *Research Quarterly for Exercise and Sport* 64 (December 1993): 365–76.

Blessing, D. L. "The Energy Cost of Bench Stepping with and Without One and Two Pound Hand-Held Weights." *Medicine and Science in Sports and Exercise* 23 (No. 4, 1991): S28 (abstract).

Borg, G. A. V. "Psychophysical Bases of Perceived Exertion." *Medicine and Science in Sports and Exercise* 14 (No. 5, 1982): 377–81.

Boyer, J. L. "Effects of Chronic Exercise on Cardiovascular Function." *Physical Fitness Research Digest* 2 (1972): 1.

Brody, J. *Jane Brody's Nutrition Book.* New York: W. W. Norton, 1981.

Brooks, G. A., and T. D. Fahey. *Exercise Physiology: Human Bioenergetics and Its Applications.* New York: John Wiley & Sons, 1984.

Brown, D. *Dawn Brown's Complete Guide to Step Aerobics.* Boston: Jones and Bartlett, 1992.

Calarco, R. M., J. Wygand, J. Kramer, M. Yoke, and F. D'Zamko. "The Metabolic Cost of Six Common Movement Patterns of Bench Step Aerobic Dance." *Medicine and Science in Sports and Exercise* 23 (No. 4, 1991): S140 (abstract).

Cassidy, C. "Should You Add a Little Weight to Your Workout?" *Women's Sports and Fitness* 8 (March 1986): 38–39, 47.

Casten, C. *Aqua Aerobics Today.* Minneapolis/St. Paul: West Publishing Co., 1994.

Cooper Institute for Aerobics Research. *The Prudential FIT-NESSGRAM Test Administration Manual.* Dallas: Cooper Institute for Aerobics Research, 1992.

Cooper, K. H. *The Aerobics Program for Total Well-Being.* New York: M. Evans, 1982.

Copeland, C., L. Francis, P. Francis, and G. Miller. *Power Step Reebok.* Boston: Reebok International, 1992.

Corbin, C. B., and R. Lindsey. *Concepts of Physical Fitness with Laboratories.* 5th ed. Dubuque, IA: Wm C Brown, 1985.

———. *Fitness for Life.* 2nd ed. Glenview, IL: Scott, Foresman, 1983.

Corbin, C. B., and M. L. Noble. "Flexibility." *Journal of Physical Education and Recreation* 51 (No. 6, 1980): 23–26; 57–60.

Couldry, W., C. B. Corbin, and A. Wilcox. "Carotid vs. Radial Pulse Counts." *The Physician and Sportsmedicine* 10 (No. 12, 1982): 67–72.

de Vries, H. A. *Physiology of Exercise.* 3rd ed. Dubuque, IA: Wm C Brown, 1980.

Dishman, R. K. "Exercise Compliance: A New View for Public Health." *The Physician and Sportsmedicine* 14 (No. 5, 1986): 127–43.

Elder, D. "Cardio Combat." *Women's Sports and Fitness* 14 (January–February 1992): 55–56.

Fahey, T. D., P. M. Insel, and W. T. Roth. *Fit and Well.* Mountain View, CA: Mayfield, 1994.

Falls, H. B. "Modern Concepts of Physical Fitness." *Journal of Physical Education and Recreation* 51 (April 1980): 25–27.

Fardy, P. S. "Isometric Exercise and the Cardiovascular System." *The Physician and Sportsmedicine* 9 (No. 9, 1981): 42.

Foster, C., D. L. Costill, and W. J. Fink. "Effects of Preexercise Feedings on Endurance Performance." *Medicine and Science in Sports* 11 (No. 1, 1979): 1–5.

Francis, L., P. Francis, and G. Miller. *Introduction to Step Reebok.* Boston: Reebok International, 1991.

Francis, L. L. "Improving Aerobic Dance Programs: The Key Role of Colleges and Universities." *Journal of Physical Education, Recreation, and Dance* 62 (September 1991): 59–62.

———. "Teaching Step Training." *Journal of Physical Education, Recreation, and Dance* 64 (March 1993): 26–30.

Garrick, J. G., D. M. Gillien, and P. Whiteside. "The Epidemiology of Aerobic Dance Injuries." *The American Journal of Sports Medicine* 14 (1986): 67–72.

Gerson, R. "Point-Counterpoint: Calisthenics Before Aerobics." *Dance Exercise Today* (May/June 1985): 26–28.

Giddens, S. "Yogarobics." *Women's Sports and Fitness* 14 (January–February 1992): 54.

Gordon, J. "Jam Up for Jelly Bellies: Street Dancing Pumps New Life into Aerobics." *Newsweek* 117 (April 29, 1991): 57.

Grant, G. *Technical Manual and Dictionary of Classical Ballet.* New York: Dover, 1967.

Harste, A. "Bench Aerobics: A Step in the Right Direction?" *The Physician and Sportsmedicine* 18 (No. 6, 1990): 25–26.

Hoeger, W. W. K., and S. A. Hoeger. *Lifetime Physical Fitness and Wellness.* 3rd ed. Englewood, CO: Morton, 1992.

Holt, L. E., T. M. Travis, and T. Okita. "Comparative Study of Three Stretching Techniques." *Perceptual and Motor Skills* 31 (1970): 611.

Hooper, P. L., and B. J. Noland. "Aerobic Dance Program Improves Cardiovascular Fitness in Men." *The Physician and Sportsmedicine* 12 (No. 5, 1984): 132–35.

Hopkins, D. R., B. Murrah, W. W. K. Hoeger, and R. C. Rhodes. "Effect of Low-Impact Aerobic Dance on the Functional Fitness of Elderly Women." *The Gerontologist* 30 (April 1990): 189–92.

Imm, P. S. "Perceived Benefits of Participants in an Employees' Aerobic Fitness Program." *Perceptual and Motor Skills* 71 (December 1990): 753–54.

International Dance-Exercise Association (IDEA) Foundation. *Aerobic Dance-Exercise Instructor Manual.* San Diego: International Dance-Exercise Association (IDEA) Foundation, 1987.

Jones, A. "Point-Counterpoint: Aerobics Before Calisthenics." *Dance Exercise Today* (May/June 1985): 27–28.

Jordan, P. *Fitness Theory and Practice.* Sherman Oaks, CA: Aerobics and Fitness Association of America, 1993.

Kannel, W. B., and P. Sorlie. "Some Health Benefits of Physical Activity: The Framingham Study." *Archives of Internal Medicine* 139 (1979): 857–61.

Karvonen, M., E. Kentala, and O. Mustalof. "The Effects of Training on Heart Rate: A Longitudinal Study." *Annales of Medicinae Experimentalis et Biologiae Fenniae* 35 (1957): 307–15.

Kernodle, R. G. "Space: The Unexplored Frontier of Aerobic Dance." *Journal of Physical Education, Recreation, and Dance* 63 (May–June 1992): 65–69.

Koszuta, L. E. "Low-Impact Aerobics: Better than Traditional Aerobic Dance?" *The Physician and Sportsmedicine* 14 (No. 6, 1986): 156–61.

Krasevec, J. A., and D. C. Grimes. *HydroRobics.* 2nd ed. West Point, NY: Leisure Press, 1985.

Kraus, H., and W. Raab. *Hypokinetic Disease.* Springfield, IL: C. C. Thomas, 1961.

Kravitz, L. "Getting in Step." *Women's Sports and Fitness* 12 (April 1993): 18.

Kravitz, L., and D. Furst. "Influence of Reward and Social Support on Exercise Adherence in Aerobic Dance Classes." *Psychological Reports* 69 (No. 2, 1991): 423–26.

Little, J. C. "The Athlete's Neurosis—A Deprivation Crisis." In *Psychology of Running,* edited by M. H. Scacks and M. L. Sachs. Champaign, IL: Human Kinetics, 1981.

MacFarlane, P. A. "Out with the Sit-Up, In with the Curl-Up." *Journal of Physical Education, Recreation, and Dance* 64 (August 1993): 62–66.

Mahurin, J., and T. P. Martin. "Anaerobic Threshold: A Trainable Component of Cardiovascular Fitness." *Motor Skills: Theory into Practice* 6 (1982): 41.

Malanka, P. "Aerobics Rebound! From Sports Drills to Step Training, New Techniques Are Transforming the Way America Works Out." *Health* 22 (March 1990): 59–65.

Martin, J. E., and P. M. Dubbert. "Adherence to Exercise." In *Exercise and Sports Sciences Review,* edited by R. J. Terjung. New York: Macmillan, 1985.

Martin, K. "Soft Aerobics: Gain Without Pain?" *Ms* 14 (May 1986): 52, 54, 113.

Mathews, D. K., and E. L. Fox. *The Physiological Basis of Physical Education and Athletics.* Philadelphia: W. B. Saunders, 1976.

McArdle, W., L. Zwiren, and J. R. Magel. "Validity of the Postexercise Heart Rate as a Means of Estimating Heart Rate During Work of Varying Intensities." *Research Quarterly* 40 (1969): 523–28.

McArdle, W. D., F. I. Katch, and V. L. Katch. *Exercise Physiology: Energy, Nutrition, and Human Performance.* Philadelphia: Lea & Febiger, 1981.

McArdle, W. D., G. S. Pechar, F. I. Katch, and J. R. Magel. "Percentile Norms for a Valid Step Test in College Women." *Research Quarterly* 44 (No. 4, 1973): 498–500.

Morrow, J. R., Jr., H. B. Falls, and H. W. Kohl III. (Eds.). *The Prudential FITNESSGRAM Technical Reference Manual.* Dallas: Cooper Institute for Aerobics Research, 1994.

Mosher, C. "Is Low-Impact High-Risk?" *Women's Sports and Fitness* 8 (April 1986): 68–69.

Multiple Risk Factor Intervention Trial Research Group. "Multiple Risk Factor Intervention Trial." *Journal of the American Medical Association* 248 (1982): 1465–77.

National Dairy Council. *Guide to Wise Food Choices.* Rosemont, IL: National Dairy Council, 1978.

National Research Council, National Academy of Sciences. *Diet and Health: Implications for Reducing Chronic Disease Risk.* Washington, D.C., 1989.

Neporent, L. "Aerobics: Watch Your Step." *Women's Sports and Fitness* 14 (September 1992): 71–72.

Nethery, V. M., and P.A. Harmer. "The Energy Cost of Slideboard Training and Cycle Ergometry." Unpublished ms. Department of Physical Education, Health Education, and Leisure Services, Central Washington University, Ellensburg, WA; and Exercise Science, Willamette University, Salem, OR, 1994.

Nieman, D. C. *The Sports Medicine Fitness Course.* Palo Alto, CA: Bull Publishing, 1986.

Olson, M. S., H. N. Wiliford, D. L. Blessing, and R. Greathouse. "Cardiorespiratory Responses to 'Aerobic' Bench Stepping Exercise in Females." *Medicine and Science in Sports and Exercise* 23 (No. 4, 1991): S27 (abstract).

Otto, R. M., C. A. Parker, T. K. Smith, J. W. Wygand, and H. R. Perez. "The Energy Cost of Low Impact and High Impact Aerobic Dance Exercise." *Medicine and Science in Sports and Exercise* 18 (No. 2, 1986): 523 (abstract).

Paffenbarger, R. S., and R. T. Hyde. "Exercise as Protection Against Heart Attack." *New England Journal of Medicine* 302 (1980): 1026.

Paffenbarger, R. S., R. T. Hyde, A. L. Wing, and C. Hsieh. "Physical Activity, All-Cause Mortality, and Longevity of College Alumni." *New England Journal of Medicine* 314 (1986): 605–13.

Paul, L. "Funky Fitness: Victoria Johnson's Technifunk Aerobics Mixes Exercise and Expressive Dance." *Women's Sports and Fitness* 14 (No. 1, 1992): 68–69.

Peterson, J. A. *Conditioning for a Purpose.* West Point, NY: Leisure Press, 1977.

Pollock, M. L. "How Much Exercise Is Enough?" *The Physician and Sportsmedicine* 6 (No. 6, 1978): 50–56; 58–60; 63–64.

Pollock, M. L., and S. N. Blair. "Analysis into Action: Exercise Prescription." *Journal of Physical Education and Recreation* 52 (No. 1, 1981): 30–35, 81.

Pollock, M. L., L. Gettman, C. Mileses, M. Bah, J. Durstine, and R. Johnson. "Effects of Frequency and Duration of Training on Attrition and Incidence of Injury." *Medicine and Science in Sports* 9 (No. 1, 1977): 31–36.

———. *Exercise in Health and Disease.* Philadelphia: W. B. Saunders, 1984.

Pollock, M. L., J. H. Wilmore, and S. M. Fox. *Health and Fitness Through Physical Activity.* New York: John Wiley & Sons, 1978.

Reebok International, Ltd. *Slide Reebok^{TM} Professional Training Manual.* Los Angeles: Reebok University Press, 1993.

Reeder, S. "The New Aerobics: Now You Can Bop to the Beat Without Jarring Your Joints." *Women's Sports and Fitness* 7 (December 1985): 27–29.

Ricci, B., M. Marchetti, and F. Figura. "Biomechanics of Sit-Up Exercises." *Medicine and Science in Sports and Exercise* 13 (No. 1, 1981): 54–59.

Richie, D. H., S. F. Kelso, and P. A. Bellucci. "Aerobic Dance Injuries: A Retrospective Study of Instructors and Participants." *The Physician and Sportsmedicine* 13 (No. 2, 1985): 134–35.

Schultz, P. "Flexibility: Day of the Static Stretch." *The Physician and Sportsmedicine* 7 (No. 11, 1979): 109–114, 117.

Segal, D. D. "An Anatomic and Biomechanic Approach to Low Back Health: A Preventive Approach." *Journal of Sports Medicine* 23 (1983): 411–21.

Shellock, F. G. "Physiological Benefits of Warm-Up." *The Physician and Sportsmedicine* 11 (No. 10, 1983): 134–39.

Shephard, R. J. "Motivation: The Key to Fitness Compliance." *The Physician and Sportsmedicine* 13 (No. 6, 1985): 88–98.

Silvestri, L., and J. Oescher. "Use of Aerobic Dance and Light Weights in Improving Measures of Strength, Endurance, and Flexibility." *Perceptual and Motor Skills* 70 (April 1990): 595–600.

Skinner, J. S., R. Hursler, V. Bergsteinova, and E. R. Buskirk. "The Validity and Reliability of a Rating Scale of Perceived Exertion." *Medicine and Science in Sports* 5 (No. 2, 1973): 94–96.

Smith, E. L. "Exercise for Prevention of Osteoporosis: A Review." *The Physician and Sportsmedicine* (No. 3, 1982): 72–83.

Smith, T. "Swing into Salsa." *Women's Sports and Fitness* 13 (March 1991): 60.

Stanforth, D., K. Velasquez, and P. R. Stanforth. "The Effect of Bench Height and Rate of Stepping on the Metabolic Cost of Bench Stepping." *Medicine and Science in Sports and Exercise* 23 (No. 4, 1991): S143 (abstract).

Thompson, C. W., and R. T. Floyd. *Manual of Structural Kinesiology.* 12th ed. St. Louis, MO: Mosby, 1994.

Thomsen, D., and D. L. Ballor. "Physiological Responses During Aerobic Dance of Individuals Grouped by Aerobic Capacity and Dance Experience." *Research Quarterly for Exercise and Sport* 62 (March 1991): 68–72.

The USDA Food Guide in "Preparing Foods and Planning Menus Using the Dietary Guidelines." *HG*, 232–38, 1989.

U.S. Department of Agriculture, U. S. Department of Human Services. *Nutrition and Your Health: Dietary Guidelines for Americans.* 3rd ed. Washington, D.C., 1990.

United States Senate Select Committee on Nutrition and Human Needs. *Dietary Goals for the United States.* 2nd ed. Washington, D.C.: U.S. Government Printing Office, 1977.

VanGalen, P. A. *Exercising with Dyna-band, Total Body Toner.* Hudson, OH: Thomas B. Gilliam Ent., Inc., 1987.

Veit, K. "Bodysculpt." *Women's Sports and Fitness.* 14 (January–February 1992): 52.

Vetter, W. L., D. L. Helfet, K. Spear, and L. S. Matthews. "Aerobic Dance Injuries." *The Physician and Sportsmedicine* 13 (No. 2, 1985): 114–20.

Vincent, W. J., and S. D. Britten. "Evaluation of the Curl-Up—A Substitute for the Bent Knee Sit-Up." *Journal of Physical Education, Recreation, and Dance* 51 (1980): 74–75.

Voelz, C. *Motivation in Coaching a Team Sport.* Washington, D.C.: National Association for Girls & Women in Sport, American Association of Physical Education and Recreation, 1976.

Watterson, V. V. "The Effects of Aerobic Dance on Cardiovascular Fitness." *The Physician and Sportsmedicine* 12 (No. 10, 1984): 138–45.

Webb, Tamilee. *Tamilee Webb's Original Rubber Band Workout.* New York: Workman Publishing, 1986.

Wells, C. L. *Women, Sport, and Performance.* Champaign, IL: Human Kinetics, 1985.

Wilson, B. R., D. C. Nirwtsu, and J. M. Lindle. "Metabolic Responses to Three Water-Aerobic Exercises." *Research Quarterly for Exercise and Sport* 63 (March 1992 Supplement): A-30.

Winters, C. "Doing the Two-Step." *American Health* 12 (May 1993): 92.

Yoxall, P. "All the Right Moves." *Current Health 2* 20 (November 1993): 16–17.

Glossary

adenosine triphosphate (ATP)   The high-energy phosphate molecule used to make cellular energy. Muscle cells use ATP to fuel contraction.

aerobic   With or in the presence of oxygen.

aerobic exercise   Exercise that demands a large and continuous supply of oxygen and that ultimately results in the improvement of the oxygen carrying and delivery systems. Exercise that involves continuous rhythmic large-muscle movements.

aerobic glycolysis   The metabolic process of breaking down carbohydrate in the presence of oxygen.

aerobic system   The metabolic processes of breaking down carbohydrate, fat, and protein in the presence of oxygen to produce energy (ATP).

aerobic target zone   The fitness target zone for aerobic activity. *See* fitness target zone.

agonist   A muscle that is undergoing contraction.

anaerobic   Without or in the absence of oxygen.

anaerobic glycolysis   The metabolic process of breaking down carbohydrate in the absence of oxygen to produce energy (ATP). (Synonym: lactic acid system)

anaerobic system   The metabolic processes that produce energy (ATP) in the absence of oxygen. *See* phosphagen system and anaerobic glycolysis.

anorexia nervosa   An eating disorder characterized by a continual desire to lose weight because of fear of being fat. Unless treated, individuals suffering from this disease can starve themselves to death.

antagonist   A muscle working in opposition to the agonist. When the agonist contracts, the antagonist relaxes.

antagonist stretching   A type of stretching where the agonist is contracted to aid the stretch and relaxation of the antagonist. Works on the principle of reciprocal innervation.

aqua aerobics   A low-impact form of aerobic conditioning performed in water using water resistance to enhance training.

arteriosclerosis   Hardening of the arteries. *See* atherosclerosis.

artery   A vessel that carries blood away from the heart.

assisted stretch   A type of stretching where the individual pulls or pushes a body part or has a partner pull or push the body part until stretch is achieved.

atherosclerosis   A specific form of arteriosclerosis characterized by the formation of fatty deposits (plaque) along the walls of the arteries.

ATP   *See* adenosine triphosphate.

ballistic stretching   A technique used to develop flexibility. It is characterized by a series of bouncing or pulsing movements that alternately stretch and then relax the muscle. These movements may elicit the stretch reflex. (Opposite of static stretching.)

blood pressure   The amount of pressure the blood exerts against the walls of the arteries during heart contraction (systolic pressure) and heart relaxation (diastolic pressure). It is generally represented as a fraction: systolic/diastolic pressure.

body composition   The relative amounts of lean body mass and fat in the body.

bpm   Beats per minute.

bulimia   An eating disorder characterized by binge-and-purge behavior. Purging may be accomplished through self-induced vomiting or use of diuretics or laxatives.

calorie   Common usage form of the word *kilocalorie*. A measure of the value of foods to produce heat and energy in the human body. One calorie is equal to the amount of heat required to raise the temperature of 1 gram of water 1 degree C.

capillaries The smallest blood vessels in the body. They supply blood (oxygen) to the tissues.

carbohydrates Compounds such as sugars and starches that are made up of carbon, hydrogen, and oxygen. Carbohydrates serve as the primary source of energy for the body. They are broken down and transported in the blood as glucose and is stored in the liver and muscles as glycogen. Dietary sources include complex carbohydrates (e.g., grains and beans) and simple carbohydrates (e.g., refined sugars and natural sugars).

cardiac output The amount of blood pumped by the heart in one minute.

cardiorespiratory endurance The ability to perform large-muscle movements over a sustained period of time. Also, the ability of the lung-heart system to deliver oxygen for sustained energy production. (Synonyms: cardiovascular fitness; cardiorespiratory endurance or fitness)

carotid artery An artery that runs close to the surface of the skin just to the side (either side) of the larynx. This artery is commonly used for counting the pulse.

CHD *See* coronary heart disease.

cholesterol A fatty substance in the blood and body tissues that is naturally synthesized by the body and is also contained in certain foods. High levels of cholesterol in the blood are associated with atherosclerosis: this is a major risk factor contributing to coronary heart disease.

circuit training A method of aerobic or resistance training that involves moving through a series of exercise stations with short or no breaks between stations.

concentric contraction A muscle contraction during which the muscle is shortening.

coronary arteries The arteries that supply the heart with oxygen.

coronary heart disease (CHD) The major form of cardiovascular disease, or a disease of the heart or blood vessels. It is the single largest leading cause of death in the United States.

diastolic pressure The pressure exerted by the blood in the arteries when the heart is filling. Diastolic pressure is represented by the denominator in the blood-pressure fraction.

duration The length of a single exercise session.

eccentric contraction A muscle contraction during which the muscle is lengthening.

EHR *See* exercise heart rate.

energy balance A state where caloric intake is equal to caloric expenditure. No weight change occurs during energy balance.

exercise heart rate (EHR) The number of times the heart beats per minute (or per ten seconds) during an exercise session.

extrinsic motivation Motivation that has its source outside the individual.

fat One of the six essential nutrients. This energy-rich compound made up of glycerol and fatty acids serves as a source of energy for the body, particularly during aerobic activity. It is stored as adipose tissue.

fatty acid oxidation An aerobic metabolic process that produces energy (ATP) through the breakdown of fatty acids.

FIT An acronym for the three variables involved in overload: frequency, intensity, and time. (Also called FITT, where the last T is type of activity.)

fitness target zone The optimal range of exercise, defined by frequency, intensity, and time (duration) and performed with the purpose of maintaining or improving physical fitness. The lower limit of the zone is called the threshold of training. The upper limit is the maximum amount of exercise that is beneficial.

flexibility The ability to move a joint through its full range of motion.

frequency The number of times a person exercises per week.

glucose The simplest form of sugar. Carbohydrate is broken down into glucose before being absorbed into the bloodstream and taken to the cell for the production of energy.

HDL *See* high-density lipoprotein.

heart rate (HR) The number of times the heart beats per minute.

heart rate reserve (HR_{max}reserve) The maximum heart rate minus the resting heart rate.

HIA *See* high-impact aerobics.

high-density lipoprotein (HDL) A complex of lipids (fat) and proteins that picks up cholesterol in the blood and carries it to the liver. Exercise increases the amount of HDL in the blood. (Often called HDL-C when carrying cholesterol.)

high-impact aerobics (HIA) A style of aerobics in which both feet may temporarily leave the floor at the same time when performing moves such as jogging, jumping, and hopping.

homeostasis State of balance or dynamic equilibrium. The energy demand is being met by energy production.

HRmax *See* maximum heart rate.

HR_{max}reserve *See* heart rate reserve.

hydrostatic weighing A method of estimating body fat. (Synonym: underwater weighing)

hypertrophy An increase in size. In exercise this usually refers to an increase in muscle size.

intensity The level of exertion during exercise.

interval training An anaerobic method of conditioning that alternates short, high-intensity exercise bouts with short rest periods.

intrinsic motivation Motivation that arises from within a person; self-motivation.

isometric contraction A muscle contraction where there is tension but no movement. It is used to increase strength in one position.

isotonic contraction A muscle contraction taken over a range of motion. It is used to increase strength throughout a movement. (Synonym: dynamic contraction)

Karvonen formula A method of calculating the intensity target range for aerobic work using a percentage of the heart rate reserve.

lactic acid A by-product of high-intensity anaerobic exercise. Accumulation of lactic acid is associated with muscle fatigue and "burn."

lactic acid system *See* anaerobic glycolysis.

LDL *See* low-density lipoprotein.

lean body mass (LBM) All the tissues of the body except fat. LBM includes bone, muscle, water, organs, connective tissue, etc., and is used to determine body composition.

LIA *See* low-impact aerobics.

ligament The fibrous tissue that connects bones to bones.

low-density lipoprotein (LDL) A complex of lipids and proteins that carries cholesterol and deposits it along the walls of the arteries. (Often called LDL-C when carrying cholesterol.) High concentrations of LDL are associated with an increased risk of heart disease.

low-impact aerobics (LIA) A type of aerobics in which the participant keeps one foot on the floor at all times. It is often characterized by moderately paced movements involving a full range of motion with a lot of upper-body work.

maximum heart rate (HRmax) The highest heart rate obtainable with exertion.

maximum heart rate formula A method of estimating the intensity range for an aerobic workout using a percentage (70 to 85 percent) of the maximum heart rate. (Synonym: zero to peak formula)

minerals Inorganic compounds that are essential to normal body function.

muscular endurance The ability of a muscle, or group of muscles, to apply force repeatedly or to sustain a muscular contraction for a period of time.

muscular strength The maximum force a muscle, or group of muscles, can exert against a resistance.

overfat A condition where the percentage of body weight that is fat weight is too high.

overweight An amount of weight above the average as determined by a standard height/weight chart.

oxygen consumption The rate at which oxygen is used to produce energy, measured in liters per minute or milliliters per kilogram of body weight per minute. (Synonym: oxygen uptake)

passive stretching A partner places a person in a stretch position. The person being stretched tries to relax the stretched muscle.

phosphagen system An anaerobic system that rapidly produces energy through the breakdown and resynthesis of high-energy phosphagens (not carbohydrate). This system can supply only a few seconds of energy.

physical fitness The physical aspects of a person's well-being that enable a person to function at an optimal level.

PNF stretching A method of stretching that uses proprioceptive neuromuscular facilitation (PNF). First the muscle is isometrically contracted, and then it is stretched.

pre-exercise heart rate (PreHR) The rate at which the heart is beating prior to exercise.

principle of individuality An exercise principle that states that any two people can react differently to the same exercise.

principle of overload An exercise principle stating that a physiological system or organ of the body repeatedly subjected to greater than normal stress will adapt to the stress. A proper amount of overload will result in positive adaptations.

principle of overuse An exercise principle that states that too much stress over a period of time can result in fatigue and injury.

principle of progression An exercise principle that states that the gradual increase (or overload) of the intensity, frequency, or duration of exercise will improve physical fitness.

principle of reversibility An exercise principle stating that a physiological system or organ that is not repeatedly stressed but is instead subjected to less than normal amounts of stress will adapt by deconditioning. (Synonym: use/disuse principle)

principle of specificity An exercise principle stating that physiological adaptations are specific to the systems that are overloaded with exercise.

protein A compound made up of amino acids that is found in certain foods. It is primarily used to build and repair body tissues but may also serve as a source of energy.

pulse The wave of pressure felt in the arteries when the heart beats.

radial artery An artery that runs close to the surface of the skin on the inside of the wrist. This artery is commonly used for counting the pulse.

rating of perceived exertion (RPE) A method of estimating the intensity of an exercise session that uses a scale of numbers with brief qualifiers developed by Borg.

recovery heart rate (RecHR) The rate at which the heart rate returns to a preexercise level following exercise.

repetition maximum To exert a maximal force over one (1RM) or more (10RM) repetitions.

resting heart rate (RHR) The rate which the heart beats at when the body is at rest.

RICE An acronym for immediate first aid for injuries such as sprains, strains, and contusions: rest, ice, compression, elevation.

RM *See* Repetition maximum.

RPE *See* rating of perceived exertion.

shinsplints A general term for pain on the front or side of the shin. A common overuse injury in aerobic activity.

skin-fold technique A method of estimating a person's percentage of body fat. Subcutaneous fat is measured using a skin-fold caliper.

slide aerobics A form of aerobic conditioning that uses a manufactured slideboard to perform predominantly lateral skating-type movements. Forward and backward movements can also be performed. (Synonym: slideboard training)

spot reducing One of the all-time greatest myths, stating that an individual can take fat off a specific part of the body by exercising that specific part. A person actually can lose fat throughout the body only by exercising aerobically and eating a proper diet.

sprain Overstretching or tearing a ligament or joint capsule, resulting in swelling, discoloration, and pain.

static stretching A technique of developing flexibility that places the muscle in a stretch position and then holds that stretch without moving. (Opposite of ballistic stretching.)

step aerobics A form of aerobic dance exercise where you step up and down on a bench to the beat of the music at a rate of 120–122 bpm.

strain Overstretching or tearing a muscle or tendon, resulting in swelling, discoloration, and pain.

strength *See* muscular strength.

stretch reflex The automatic muscular contraction that occurs when a muscle is suddenly stretched.

stroke volume The amount of blood the heart pumps in one beat.

systolic pressure The pressure exerted by the blood in the arteries when the heart is contracting. Systolic pressure is represented by the numerator in the blood pressure fraction.

target heart rate zone *See* training heart rate range.

TC *See* total cholesterol.

tendinitis Inflammation of a tendon. This is a common overuse injury.

tendon Fibrous tissue that connects muscle to bone.

THR *See* training heart rate range.

threshold of aerobic training The lower limit of the aerobic target zone. It is usually described by a percentage of the maximum volume of oxygen consumed, the maximum heart rate, or the heart rate reserve. *See* threshold of training.

threshold of training The minimum amount and intensity of exercise that must be performed for an individual to make physical fitness gains.

time The length of a single exercise session.

total cholesterol The sum of HDL and LDL.

training heart rate range (THR) The optimum intensity range for aerobic exercise using the exercise heart rate as the indicator of intensity. Training within the range improves cardiorespiratory endurance. (Synonym: target heart rate zone)

underwater weighing *See* hydrostatic weighing.

use/disuse principle *See* principle of reversibility.

vein A vessel that carries blood toward the heart.

venous pump Action of the muscles that helps to massage blood up the veins against gravity.

vitamins Organic compounds that help release energy from food and act as metabolic regulators. Vitamins A, D, E, and K are fat soluble; the rest are water soluble.

VO$_2$max The largest amount of oxygen the body can consume in one minute, measured in liters per minute or milliliters per kilogram of body weight per minute. (Synonym: maximum oxygen uptake or MOU)

warm-up The period of time in which individuals prepare the body for vigorous activity by performing easy movements through a range of motion, thus raising the core temperature of the body and stretching out and lubricating muscles and joints. Leading into the aerobic workout is a gradual increase in activity level that allows the heart and lungs to make a smooth transition into exercise.

water aerobics *See* aqua aerobics.

wellness Taking control of your personal well-being, including mental, social, physical, intellectual, environmental, and spiritual health.

zero to peak formula *See* maximum heart rate formula.

APPENDIX

MUSCLES OF THE BODY

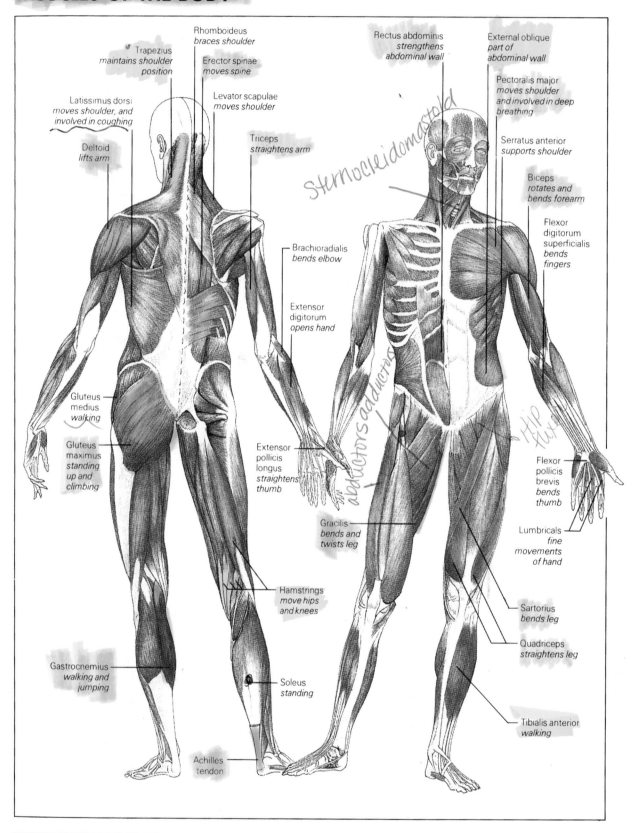

Trapezius
maintains shoulder position

Rhomboideus
braces shoulder

Erector spinae
moves spine

Levator scapulae
moves shoulder

Latissimus dorsi
moves shoulder, and involved in coughing

Deltoid
lifts arm

Triceps
straightens arm

Brachioradialis
bends elbow

Extensor digitorum
opens hand

Gluteus medius
walking

Gluteus maximus
standing up and climbing

Extensor pollicis longus
straightens thumb

Gracilis
bends and twists leg

Hamstrings
move hips and knees

Gastrocnemius
walking and jumping

Soleus
standing

Achilles tendon

Rectus abdominis
strengthens abdominal wall

External oblique
part of abdominal wall

Pectoralis major
moves shoulder and involved in deep breathing

Serratus anterior
supports shoulder

Biceps
rotates and bends forearm

Flexor digitorum superficialis
bends fingers

Flexor pollicis brevis
bends thumb

Lumbricals
fine movements of hand

Sartorius
bends leg

Quadriceps
straightens leg

Tibialis anterior
walking

From: *The American Medical Association Family Medical Guide* by American Medical Association. Copyright © 1982 by the American Medical Association. Reprinted with permission of Random House, Inc.

YOUR BACK AND HOW TO CARE FOR IT

Your back and how to care for it

Whatever the cause of low back pain, part of its treatment is the correction of faulty posture. But good posture is not simply a matter of "standing tall." It refers to correct use of the body at all times. In fact, for the body to function in the best of health it must be so used that no strain is put upon muscles, joints, bones, and ligaments. To prevent low back pain, avoiding strain must become a way of life, practiced while lying, sitting, standing, walking, working, and exercising. When body position is correct, internal organs have enough room to function normally and blood circulates more freely.

With the help of this guide, you can begin to correct the positions and movements which bring on or aggravate backache. Particular attention should be paid to the positions recommended for resting, since it is possible to strain the muscles of the back and neck even while lying in bed. By learning to live with good posture, under all circumstances, you will gradually develop the proper carriage and stronger muscles needed to protect and support your hard-working back.

HOW TO STAY ON YOUR FEET WITHOUT TIRING YOUR BACK
To prevent strain and pain in everyday activities, it is restful to change from one task to another before fatigue sets in. Housewives can lie down between chores; others should check body position frequently, drawing in the abdomen, flattening the back, bending the knees slightly.

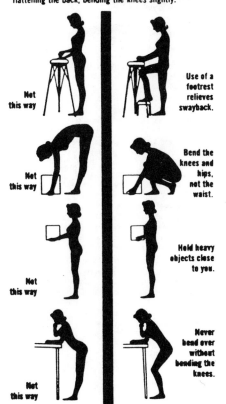

Not this way / **Not this way** / **Not this way** / **Not this way**

Use of a footrest relieves swayback.
Bend the knees and hips, not the waist.
Hold heavy objects close to you.
Never bend over without bending the knees.

CHECK YOUR CARRIAGE HERE
In correct, fully erect posture, a line dropped from the ear will go through the tip of the shoulder, middle of hip, back of kneecap, and front of anklebone.

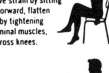

Incorrect: Lower back is arched or hollow.
Incorrect: Upper back is stooped, lower back is arched, abdomen sags.

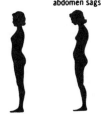

Incorrect: Note how, in strained position, pelvis tilts forward, chin is out, and ribs are down, crowding internal organs.
Correct: In correct position, chin is in, head up, back flattened, pelvis held straight.

To find the correct standing position: Stand one foot away from wall. Now sit against wall, bending knees slightly. Tighten abdominal and buttock muscles. This will tilt the pelvis back and flatten the lower spine. Holding this position, inch up the wall to standing position, by straightening the legs. Now walk around the room, maintaining the same posture. Place back against wall again to see if you have held it.

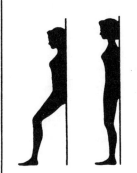

HOW TO SIT CORRECTLY
A back's best friend is a straight, hard chair. If you can't get the chair you prefer, learn to sit properly on whatever chair you get. To correct sitting position from forward slump: Throw head well back, then bend it forward to pull in the chin. This will straighten the back. Now tighten abdominal muscles to raise the chest. Check position frequently.

Relieve strain by sitting well forward, flatten back by tightening abdominal muscles, and cross knees.

Use of footrest relieves swayback. Aim is to have knees higher than hips.

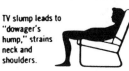

Correct way to sit while driving, close to pedals. Use seat belt or hard backrest, available commercially.

TV slump leads to "dowager's hump," strains neck and shoulders.

If chair is too high, swayback is increased.

Keep neck and back in as straight a line as possible with the spine. Bend forward from hips.

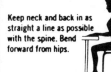

Driver's seat too far from pedals emphasizes curve in lower back.

Strained reading position. Forward thrusting strains muscles of neck and head.

(continued)

Continued.

HOW TO PUT YOUR BACK TO BED

For proper bed posture, a firm mattress is essential. Bedboards, sold commercially, or devised at home, may be used with soft mattresses. Bedboards, preferably, should be made of ¾ inch plywood. Faulty sleeping positions intensify swayback and result not only in backache but in numbness, tingling, and pain in arms and legs.

Incorrect:	Correct:
Lying flat on back makes swayback worse.	Lying on side with knees bent effectively flattens the back. Flat pillow may be used to support neck, especially when shoulders are broad.

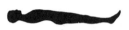

| Use of high pillow strains neck, arms, shoulders. | Sleeping on back is restful and correct when knees are properly supported. |

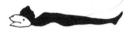
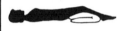

| Sleeping face down exaggerates swayback, strains neck and shoulders. | Raise the foot of the mattress eight inches to discourage sleeping on the abdomen. |

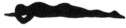

| Bending one hip and knee does not relieve swayback. | Proper arrangement of pillows for resting or reading in bed. |

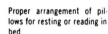

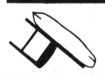

A straight-back chair used behind a pillow makes a serviceable backrest.

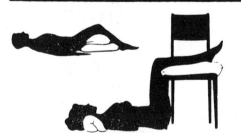

WHEN DOING NOTHING, DO IT RIGHT

Rest is the first rule for the tired, painful back. The following positions relieve pain by taking all pressure and weight off the back and legs.

Note pillows under knees to relieve strain on spine.

For complete relief and relaxing effect, these positions should be maintained from 5 to 25 minutes.

EXERCISE—WITHOUT GETTING OUT OF BED
Exercises to be performed while lying in bed are aimed not so much at strengthening muscles as at teaching correct positioning. But muscles used correctly become stronger and in time are able to support the body with the least amount of effort.

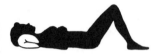

Do all exercises in this position. Legs should not be straightened.

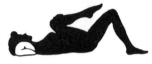

Bring knee up to chest. Lower slowly but do not straighten leg. Relax. Repeat with each leg 10 times.

Bring both knees slowly up to chest. Tighten muscles of abdomen, press back flat against bed. Hold knees to chest 20 seconds, then lower slowly. Relax. Repeat 5 times. This exercise gently stretches the shortened muscles of the lower back, while strengthening abdominal muscles. Clasp knees, bring them up to chest, at the same time coming to a sitting position. Rock back and forth.

EXERCISE—WITHOUT ATTRACTING ATTENTION
Use these inconspicuous exercises whenever you have a spare moment during the day, both to relax tension and improve the tone of important muscle groups.
1. Rotate shoulders, forward and backward.
2. Turn head slowly side to side.
3. Watch an imaginary plane take off, just below the right shoulder. Stretch neck, follow it slowly as it moves up, around and down, disappearing below the other shoulder. Repeat, starting on left side.
4. Slowly, slowly, touch left ear to left shoulder; right ear to right shoulder. Raise both shoulders to touch ears, drop them as far down as possible.
5. At any pause in the day—waiting for an elevator to arrive, for a specific traffic light to change—pull in abdominal muscles, tighten, hold it for the count of eight without breathing. Relax slowly. Increase the count gradually after the first week, practice breathing normally with the abdomen flat and contracted. Do this sitting, standing, and walking.

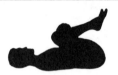

RULES TO LIVE BY—FROM NOW ON

1. Never bend from the waist only; bend the hips and knees.
2. Never lift a heavy object higher than your waist.
3. Always turn and face the object you wish to lift.
4. Avoid carrying unbalanced loads; hold heavy objects close to your body.
5. Never carry anything heavier than you can manage with ease.
6. Never lift or move heavy furniture. Wait for someone to do it who knows the principles of leverage.
7. Avoid sudden movements, sudden "overloading" of muscles. Learn to move deliberately, swinging the legs from the hips.
8. Learn to keep the head in line with the spine, when standing, sitting, lying in bed.
9. Put soft chairs and deep couches on your "don't sit" list. During prolonged sitting, cross your legs to rest your back.
10. Your doctor is the only one who can determine when low back pain is due to faulty posture. He is the best judge of when you may do general exercises for physical fitness. When you do, omit any exercise which arches or overstrains the lower back: backward bends, or forward bends, touching the toes with the knees straight.
11. Wear shoes with moderate heels, all about the same height. Avoid changing from high to low heels.
12. Put a footrail under the desk, and a footrest under the crib.
13. Diaper the baby sitting next to him or her on the bed.
14. Don't stoop and stretch to hang the wash; raise the clothesbasket and lower the washline.
15. Beg or buy a rocking chair. Rocking rests the back by changing the muscle groups used.
16. Train yourself vigorously to use your abdominal muscles to flatten your lower abdomen. In time, this muscle contraction will become habitual, making you the envied possessor of a youthful body-profile!
17. Don't strain to open windows or doors.
18. For good posture, concentrate on strengthening "nature's corset"—the abdominal and buttock muscles. The pelvic roll exercise is especially recommended to correct the postural relation between the pelvis and the spine.

SCHERING CORPORATION • KENILWORTH, N.J.

PRINTED IN U.S.A.   CE 904 11656000 6 76

WORKSHEETS

WORKSHEET 2: SUMMARY RECORD SHEET

Name: _____ Age: _____

Height: _____ Weight: _____ Healthy Weight: _____

THR: _____ beats/minute, _____ beats/10 seconds   % Fat: _____

Fitness Goals:

1.

2.

3.

Cardiovascular Fitness and Flexibility Tests

	Date _____	Date _____	Date _____
Step Test (16 1/4 inch)			
RecHR:	_____	_____	_____
Percentile Rank:	_____	_____	_____
Predicted VO$_2$max:	_____	_____	_____
Step Test (12 inch)			
RecHR:	_____	_____	_____
Fitness Rating:	_____	_____	_____
12-Minute Walk/Run			
Distance:	_____	_____	_____
Fitness Rating:	_____	_____	_____
1.5-Mile Run			
Time:	_____	_____	_____
Fitness Rating:	_____	_____	_____
Sit and Reach			
Score (cm):	_____	_____	_____
Fitness Rating:	_____	_____	_____

Five Pass/Fail Flexibility Tests (Mark "P" for pass, "F" for fail.)

	Date _____	Date _____	Date _____
Hamstring Stretch:	R _____ L _____	R _____ L _____	R _____ L
Quadriceps Stretch:	R _____ L _____	R _____ L _____	R _____ L _____
Hip Flexor Stretch:	R _____ L _____	R _____ L _____	R _____ L _____
Calf Stretch:	R _____ L _____	R _____ L _____	R _____ L _____
Lower Back Stretch:	_____	_____	_____

(continued)

Muscular Endurance Tests

Date _____   Date _____   Date _____

Curl-Ups

Number Completed: _____   _____   _____

Fitness Rating: _____   _____   _____

Push-Ups

Number Completed: _____   _____   _____

Fitness Rating: _____   _____   _____

Body Measurements

Date _____   _____Date   _____Date

Women:

Ankle (optional): R _____ L _____   R _____ L _____   R _____ L _____

Calf: R _____ L _____   R _____ L _____   R _____ L _____

Thigh: R _____ L _____   R _____ L _____   R _____ L _____

Buttocks: _____   _____   _____

Hips: _____   _____   _____

Waist: _____   _____   _____

Chest: _____   _____   _____

Upper Arm: R _____ L _____   R _____ L _____   R _____ L _____

Men:

Ankle (optional): R _____ L _____   R _____ L _____   R _____ L _____

Calf: R _____ L _____   R _____ L _____   R _____ L _____

Thigh: R _____ L _____   R _____ L _____   R _____ L _____

Buttocks: _____   _____   _____

Abdomen: _____   _____   _____

Chest (relaxed): _____   _____   _____

Chest (expanded): _____   _____   _____

Upper Arm (relaxed): R _____ L _____   R _____ L _____   R _____ L _____

Upper Arm (flexed): R _____ L _____   R _____ L _____   R _____ L _____

Shoulders: _____   _____   _____

Neck (optional): _____   _____   _____

Skin-Fold Measurements

Date _____   Date _____   Date _____

Site: _____   _____mm   _____mm   _____mm

Site: _____   _____mm   _____mm   _____mm

Site: _____   _____mm   _____mm   _____mm

TOTAL: _____mm   _____mm   _____mm

BODY FAT: _____%   _____%   _____%

WORKSHEET 3A: CALCULATING YOUR TARGET HEART RATE RANGE

Maximum Heart Rate Formula (Zero to Peak Formula)

(Refer to Chapter 3, pages 17–18.)

Step One:

Find your maximum heart rate (HRmax).

```
      220
  _____
  |      |   (your age)
- |_____|
  _____
  |      |   (HRmax)
  |_____|
```

Example:
```
    220
  -  20
  -----
    200
```

Step Two:

Find the lower end of your THR in beats/minute.

```
  _____
  |      |   (HRmax)
  |_____|
  x 0.70
  _____
  |      |   beats/minute
  |_____|
```

Example:
```
      200
  x  0.70
  -------
   140.00
```

Step Three:

Find the upper end of your THR in beats/minute.

```
  _____
  |      |   (HRmax)
  |_____|
  x 0.85
  _____
  |      |   beats/minute
  |_____|
```

Example:
```
      200
  x  0.85
  -------
     1000
     1600
  -------
   170.00
```

My target heart rate range is _____ to _____ beats/minute.
                              (lower)   (upper)

(continued)

Step Four:

Find the lower end of your THR in beats/10 seconds.

$$
6 \overline{\big)\; \boxed{\begin{array}{c} \\ \text{Step 2 Answer} \end{array}}}
$$

= _____ beats/10 seconds

Example:

```
        23.3
   6 ) 140.0
       12
       ──
        20
        18
       ──
        20
```

Step Five:

Find the upper end of your THR in beats/10 seconds.

$$
6 \overline{\big)\; \boxed{\begin{array}{c} \\ \text{Step 3 Answer} \end{array}}}
$$

= _____ beats/10 second

My target heart rate range is _____ to _____ beats/10 seconds.
(lower)   (upper)

```
        28.3
   6 ) 170.0
       12
       ──
        50
        48
       ──
        20
        18
       ──
         2
```

WORKSHEET 3B: CALCULATING YOUR TARGET HEART RATE RANGE

Karvonen Formula

(Refer to Chapter 3, pages 17–19.)

First find your average resting heart rate by counting your pulse for one minute while you are still lying in bed. Do this on three consecutive mornings.

Resting heart rate on the 1st morning: _____ beats/minute

Resting heart rate on the 2nd morning: _____ beats/minute

Resting heart rate on the 3rd morning: _____ beats/minute

Average Resting Heart Rate (RHR): _____ beats/minute

Steps One and Two:

Find your maximum heart rate and heart rate reserve.

220

– ☐ (your age)

☐ (HRmax)

– ☐ (RHR)

☐ (HR_{max}reserve)

Example:

A 20 year old with an
RHR of 50.

$$
\begin{array}{r}
220 \\
-\ 20 \\
\hline
200 \\
-\ 75 \\
\hline
125
\end{array}
$$

Steps Three and Four:

For the lower limit of the THR, calculate 60 percent of the HR_{max}reserve and add the RHR to the answer.

☐ (HR_{max}reserve)

x 0.60

☐

+ ☐ (RHR)

☐ Lower end of THR
in beats/minute

Example:

$$
\begin{array}{r}
125 \\
\times\ 0.60 \\
\hline
75.00 \\
+\ 75.00 \\
\hline
150.00
\end{array}
$$

(continued)

Steps Five and Six:

For the upper limit of the THR, calculate 80 percent of the HR_{max}reserve and add the RHR to the answer.

Example:

$$
\begin{array}{r}
125 \\
\times\ 0.80 \\
\hline
100.00 \\
+\ 75.00 \\
\hline
175.00
\end{array}
$$

$\boxed{}$ (HR_{max}reserve)

$\times\ 0.80$

$\boxed{}$

$+$ $\boxed{}$ (RHR)

$\boxed{}$ Upper end of THR in beats/minute

My target heart rate range is _____ to _____ beats/minute.
  (lower)   (upper)

Steps Seven and Eight:

Divide both ends of the THR in beats/minute by 6 to obtain a THR in beats per 10 seconds.

Example:

$$
\begin{array}{r}
25.0 \\
6\overline{)150.0} \\
12 \\
\hline
30 \\
30 \\
\hline
0
\end{array}
$$

Example:

$$
\begin{array}{r}
29.1 \\
6\overline{)175.0} \\
12 \\
\hline
55 \\
54 \\
\hline
10 \\
6 \\
\hline
4
\end{array}
$$

$6\sqrt{\boxed{}}$ $=$ $\boxed{}$
(lower limit)

$6\sqrt{\boxed{}}$ $=$ $\boxed{}$
(upper limit)

My target heart rate range is _____ to _____ beats/10 seconds.
  (lower)   (upper)

WORKSHEET 4: HEART RATE CHART

Directions:

1. On the other side of this worksheet, draw two thick horizontal lines on the graph to represent the lower and upper limits of your THR.

2. Prior to exercise, take your PreHR and plot it on the chart.

3. During aerobic exercise, take your EHR several times. Plot the highest one.

4. One minute after the aerobic portion of class, take and plot your RecHR.

5. To see heart rate trends, connect all the PreHR dots, connect all the EHR dots, and connect all the RecHR dots. (See Table 3.2 on page 21 for an example of this procedure.)

6. Each month take your RHR three mornings in a row and record the average rate in beats per minute.

Month	RHR 1	RHR 2	RHR 3	Average
1. _____	_____	_____	_____	_____
2. _____	_____	_____	_____	_____
3. _____	_____	_____	_____	_____
4. _____	_____	_____	_____	_____
5. _____	_____	_____	_____	_____
6. _____	_____	_____	_____	_____

(continued)

Heart Rate Chart

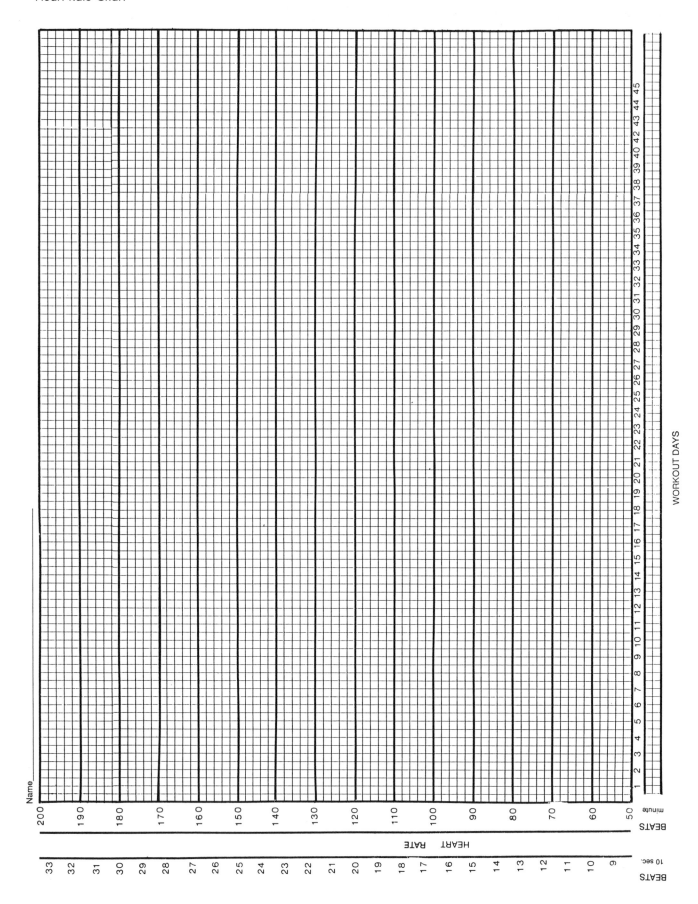

WORKSHEET 5A: CARDIORESPIRATORY FITNESS
Step Test (16 1/4 inch)

Equipment:

1. bench 16 1/4" high—a standard gymnasium bleacher

2. stopwatch

3. metronome or other means of establishing the cadence

4. pencil or pen

Directions:

1. Practice taking your heart rate. If you will be working with a partner, practice taking your partner's heart rate.

2. Warm up and stretch.

3. Face the bleachers (bench) and practice the stepping pattern: Up, Up, Down, Down.
   Up   —step up on the bench with your right foot.
   Up   —bring your left foot up on the bench.
   Down—step down to the floor with your right foot.
   Down—bring the left foot down to the floor.

4. Rest until your breathing is back to normal.

5. Set the cadence (rate at which you will step):
   women—88 beats/minute (22 step cycles/minute)
   men   —96 beats/minute (24 step cycles/minute)

6. With the start of the stopwatch begin the stepping pattern and continue stepping for 3 minutes. If you cannot complete the whole 3 minutes (too tired to keep cadence), stop and record the amount of time you were able to complete: _____ minutes _____ seconds.

7. Stop and find your pulse. Begin counting the pulse within 5 seconds after you stop stepping. Count for 15 seconds.

8. Multiply your pulse count by 4 to get beats per minute. This number is your recovery heart rate in beats/minute.
   _____ (pulse) x 4 = _____ RecHR in beats/minute

9. Look at the chart on the next page to determine your percentile ranking and predicted VO_2max. (The higher the percentile, the better your score.)
   _____ percentile ranking   _____ VO_2max

10. Stretch your legs to prevent muscle soreness.

(continued)

Percentile rankings for recovery heart rate (hr) and predicted maximal oxygen consumption for male and female college students.

PERCENTILE RANKING	RECOVERY HR FEMALE	PREDICTED MAX VO$_2$ (ML · KG^1 · MIN^1)	RECOVERY HR MALE	PREDICTED MAX VO$_2$ (ML · KG^1 · MIN^{-1})
100	128	42.2	120	60.9
95	140	40.0	124	59.3
90	148	38.5	128	57.6
85	152	37.7	136	54.2
80	156	37.0	140	52.5
75	158	36.6	144	50.9
70	160	36.3	148	49.2
65	162	35.9	149	48.8
60	163	35.7	152	47.5
55	164	35.5	154	46.7
50	166	35.1	156	45.8
45	168	34.8	160	44.1
40	170	34.4	162	43.3
35	171	34.2	164	42.5
30	172	34.0	166	41.6
25	176	33.3	168	40.8
20	180	32.6	172	39.1
15	182	32.2	176	37.4
10	184	31.8	178	36.6
5	196	29.6	184	34.1

From: W. D. McArdle, F. I. Katch, and V. L. Katch, *Exercise Physiology: Energy, Nutrition, and Human Performance.* (Philadelphia: Lea & Febiger, 1981).

WORKSHEET 5B: CARDIORESPIRATORY FITNESS
Step Test (12 inch)

Equipment:

1. bench 12" high—a step aerobics bench will work

2. stopwatch

3. metronome or other means of establishing the cadence

4. pencil or pen

Directions:

1. Practice taking your heart rate. If you will be working with a partner, practice taking your partner's heart rate.

2. Warm up and stretch.

3. Face the bench and practice the stepping pattern: Up, Up, Down, Down.
Up   —step up on the bench with your right foot.
Up   —bring your left foot up on the bench.
Down—step down to the floor with your right foot.
Down—step down to the floor with your left foot.

4. Rest until your breathing is back to normal.

5. Set the cadence (rate at which you will step) to 96 beats/minute (24 step/cycles per minute).

6. With the start of the stopwatch begin the stepping pattern and continue stepping for 3 minutes. If you cannot complete the whole 3 minutes (too tired to keep cadence), stop and record the amount of time you were able to complete: _____ minutes _____ seconds.

7. Stop and find your pulse. Begin counting the pulse within 5 seconds after you stop stepping. Count for an *entire minute.*
_____ recovery heart rate (RecHR) in beats/minute

8. Look at the chart below to determine your fitness rating.
_____ fitness rating

9. Stretch your legs to prevent muscle soreness.

Kasch 3-minute step test.

FITNESS RATING	AGE (YEARS)			
	18–26		27–60	
	M	F	M	F
Superior	68	73	69	74
Excellent	69–75	74–82	70–78	75–83
Good	76–83	83–90	79–87	84–92
Average	84–92	91–100	88–99	93–103
Fair	93–99	101–107	100–107	104–112
Poor	100–106	108–114	108–115	113–121
Very Poor	107	115	116	122

WORKSHEET 5C: CARDIORESPIRATORY FITNESS
12-Minute Walking/Running Test

Note: This is a maximum-effort test. It is recommended that you exercise regularly for 6 to 8 weeks prior to taking this test.

Equipment:

1. stopwatch

2. track or other measured course

3. pencil or pen

Directions:

1. Warm up with light jogging and stretching.

2. Run/walk as far as possible in 12 minutes. This is best achieved by maintaining a steady pace. Be sure to keep track of how far you run. You may want to do this with a partner so that you can count laps for each other.

3. Record the distance you covered: _____ miles.

4. Cool down with light jogging and stretching.

5. Consult the chart below to determine your fitness rating: _____ fitness rating.

Distance (miles) covered in 12-minute walking/running test.

FITNESS CATEGORY		AGE (YEARS)					
		13–19	20–29	30–39	40–49	50–59	60+
I. Very Poor	(men)	<1.30*	<1.22	<1.18	<1.14	<1.03	< .87
	(women)	<1.0	< .96	< .94	< .88	< .84	< .78
II. Poor	(men)	1.30–1.37	1.22–1.31	1.18–1.30	1.14–1.24	1.03–1.16	.87–1.02
	(women)	1.00–1.18	.96–1.11	.95–1.05	.88– .98	.84– .93	.78– .86
III. Fair	(men)	1.38–1.56	1.32–1.49	1.31–1.45	1.25–1.39	1.17–1.30	1.03–1.20
	(women)	1.19–1.29	1.12–1.22	1.06–1.18	.99–1.11	.94–1.05	.87– .98
IV. Good	(men)	1.57–1.72	1.50–1.64	1.46–1.56	1.40–1.53	1.31–1.44	1.21–1.32
	(women)	1.30–1.43	1.23–1.34	1.19–1.29	1.12–1.24	1.06–1.18	.99–1.09
V. Excellent	(men)	1.73–1.86	1.65–1.76	1.57–1.69	1.54–1.65	1.45–1.58	1.33–1.55
	(women)	1.44–1.51	1.35–1.45	1.30–1.39	1.25–1.34	1.19–1.30	1.10–1.18
VI. Superior	(men)	>1.87	>1.77	>1.70	>1.66	>1.59	>1.56
	(women)	>1.52	>1.46	>1.40	>1.35	>1.31	>1.19

*< Means "less than"; > means "more than."

Source: "12-Minute Walk/Run Test" from *The Aerobics Program for Total Well-Being* by Kenneth H. Cooper, M.D., M.P.H. ©1982 by Kenneth H. Cooper. Used by permission of Bantam Books, a division of Bantam Doubleday Dell Publishing Group, Inc.

WORKSHEET 5D: CARDIORESPIRATORY FITNESS
1.5-Mile Timed Run Test

Note: This is a maximum-effort test. It is recommended that you exercise regularly for 6 to 8 weeks prior to taking this test.

Equipment:

1. stopwatch

2. measured course

3. pencil or pen

Directions:

1. Warm up and stretch.

2. On the start signal, run/walk the 1.5-mile course as quickly as possible. (An even pace throughout the course is recommended.)

3. Check your time at the end of the course: _____ minutes.

4. Consult the chart below to find your fitness rating: _____ fitness rating.

Time in minutes for 1.5-mile run test.

FITNESS CATEGORY		AGE (YEARS)					
		13–19	**20–29**	**30–39**	**40–49**	**50–59**	**60+**
I. Very Poor	(men)	>15:31*	>16:01	>16:31	>17:31	>19:01	>20:01
	(women)	>18:31	>19:01	>19:31	>20:01	>20:31	>21:01
II. Poor	(men)	12:11–15:30	14:01–16:00	14:44–16:30	15:36–17:30	17:01–19:00	19:01–20:00
	(women)	16:55–18:30	18:31–19:00	19:01–19:30	19:31–20:00	20:01–20:30	20:31–21:00
III. Fair	(men)	10:49–12:10	12:01–14:00	12:31–14:45	13:01–15:35	14:31–17:00	16:16–19:00
	(women)	14:31–16:54	15:55–18:30	16:31–19:00	17:31–19:30	19:01–20:00	19:31–20:30
IV. Good	(men)	9:41–10:48	10:46–12:00	11:01–12:30	11:31–13:00	12:31–14:30	14:00–16:15
	(women)	12:30–14:30	13:31–15:54	14:31–16:30	15:56–17:30	16:31–19:00	17:31–19:30
V. Excellent	(men)	8:37– 9:40	9:45–10:45	10:00–11:00	10:30–11:30	11:00–12:30	11:15–13:59
	(women)	11:50–12:29	12:30–13:30	13:00–14:30	13:45–15:55	14:30–16:30	16:30–17:30
VI. Superior	(men)	< 8:37	< 9:45	<10:00	<10:30	<11:00	<11:15
	(women)	<11:50	<12:30	<13:00	<13:45	<14:30	<16:30

*< Means "less than"; > means "more than."

Source: "1.5 Mile Run Test" from *The Aerobics Program for Total Well-Being* by Kenneth H. Cooper, M.D., M.P.H. ©1982 by Kenneth H. Cooper. Used by permission of Bantam Books, a division of Bantam Doubleday Dell Publishing Group, Inc.

WORKSHEET 6A: FLEXIBILITY
Sit-and-Reach Test

Note: You should perform a warm-up that includes static stretching of the lower back and posterior thighs prior to taking this test. Be sure to take this test under the same conditions each time you take it. For example, if you take it the first time before working out in the afternoon, take it again at the same time of day and do it before you exercise.

Equipment:

Note: If a flexometer is available, use it. The following description assumes that one is not available.

1. meter stick

2. two partners

3. pencil or pen

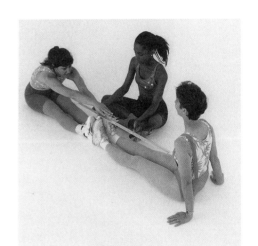

Directions:

1. Sit on the floor with your knees fully extended in front of you and your feet shoulder width apart. Have another person sit opposite you in the same position so that the soles of your feet are against those of the other person. All toes should point directly toward the ceiling throughout the test.

2. The measurer (third person) holds the meter stick so that the number 25 cm is at the bottom of the soles of your shoes. Number 1 on the meter stick should be close to you, number 39 away from you.

3. Place one hand over the other and lean forward, gently sliding your hands down the meter stick. Use a smooth, sustained motion. Do this twice.

4. The measurer will note the farthest point your fingertips reach along the meter stick. (Do not count long fingernails.) Round scores to the nearest centimeter.

5. Record your highest score: _____ cm.

6. Consult the chart below to determine your fitness rating: _____ fitness rating.

Norms by age groups and gender for trunk forward flexion (cm).*

FITNESS RATING	AGE (YEARS)											
	15–19		20–29		30–39		40–49		50–59		60–69	
	M	F	M	F	M	F	M	F	M	F	M	F
Excellent	≥39	≥43	≥40	≥41	≥38	≥41	≥35	≥38	≥35	≥39	≥33	≥35
Above Average	34–38	38–42	34–39	37–40	33–37	36–40	29–34	34–37	28–34	33–38	25–32	31–34
Average	29–33	34–37	30–33	33–36	28–32	32–35	24–28	30–33	24–27	30–32	20–24	27–30
Below Average	24–28	29–33	25–29	28–32	23–27	27–31	18–23	25–29	16–23	25–29	15–19	23–26
Poor	≤23	≤28	≤24	≤27	≤22	≤26	≤17	≤24	≤15	≤24	≤14	≤23

*Based on data from the Canada Fitness Survey, 1981.

From: *The Canadian Standardized Test of Fitness—Operations Manual*, 3rd Edition, 1986. Used with permission from the Canadian Society for Exercise Physiology in cooperation with Fitness Canada–Health Canada.

. . . .

WORKSHEET 6B: FLEXIBILITY
Five Pass/Fail Flexibility Tests

Note: These five tests are quick and easy and require no equipment. Work with a partner so that you can check each other's positions.

Note: Flexibility increases when the muscles are warm. Perform a warm-up that includes a core warm-up and static stretching of the front and back of the legs, the calves, the hip flexors, and the lower back. Repeat tests should be taken under the same conditions as the first test.

1. **Hamstring Test**
   Position: Lie flat on your back with your legs extended along the floor.
   Action: Lift one leg up.
   Pass: Lift the leg until it is perpendicular to the floor. Both knees must be straight.
   Fail: Inability to reach the perpendicular position or bending either knee.

   Score: right leg: _____ pass _____ fail

                left leg: _____ pass _____ fail

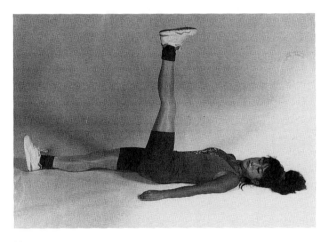

Hamstring test—pass

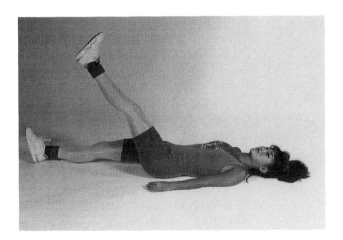

Hamstring test—fail

(continued)

2. Quadriceps Test

Position: Lie on your stomach, legs extended.

Action: Flex one leg at the knee. Grasp the ankle with your hand on the same side. Gently pull your heel to the back of your thigh. Keep the knees close together.

Pass: Touch the heel to the back of your leg with your knees close together, pulling gently on ankle or not at all.

Fail: Inability to touch heel to leg or pulling hard on the ankle.

Score: right leg: _____ pass _____ fail

left leg: _____ pass _____ fail

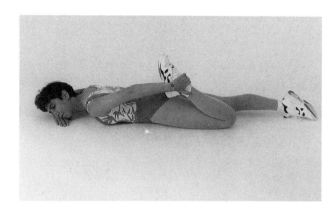

Quadriceps test—pass

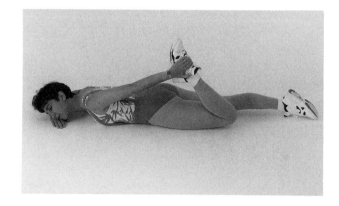

Quadriceps test—fail

3. Hip Flexor Test

Position: Lie on your back, legs straight and flat on floor.

Action: Draw one knee up to your chest. Grasp leg underneath the knee with both hands.

Pass: Touch the knee to your shoulder or lay your thigh flat along your torso, pulling gently or not at all. The other leg must remain straight.

Fail: Inability to touch knee to shoulder or lie thigh flat along torso, pulling hard on knee, or bending the other leg.

Score: right leg: _____ pass _____ fail

left leg: _____ pass _____ fail

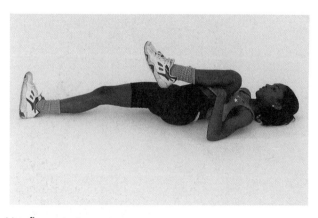

Hip flexor test—pass

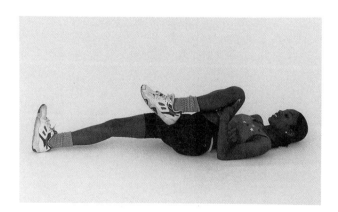

Hip flexor test—fail

(continued)

4. Lower Back Test

Position: Lie on your back with both knees bent and feet off the floor, head and lower back touching the floor.

Action: Grasp your legs underneath your knees and pull gently toward your shoulders.

Pass: Touch both knees to their respective shoulders or lay your thighs flat along your torso with lower back and head still touching the floor.

Fail: Inability to touch knees to shoulders or lay them flat along your torso, pulling hard on your knees, or lower back or head lifting from the floor.

Score: both legs: _____ pass _____ fail

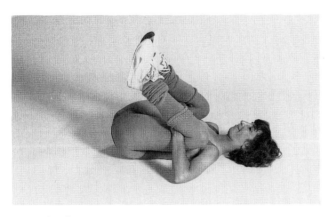

Lower back test—pass

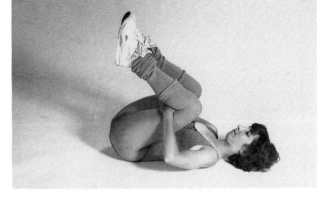

Lower back test—fail

5. Calf Test

Position: Sit on the floor with your legs extended straight out in front of you. You may place your hands behind your buttocks for support.

Action: Flex one foot. (Bring toe toward knee.)

Pass: Create a 70-degree angle between your foot and your shin.

Fail: Inability to flex far enough to create the 70-degree angle.

Score: right calf: _____ pass _____ fail

left calf: _____ pass _____ fail

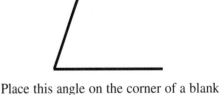

Place this angle on the corner of a blank piece of paper and extend the lines. Then hold the angle behind your partner's feet as shown in the figures below.

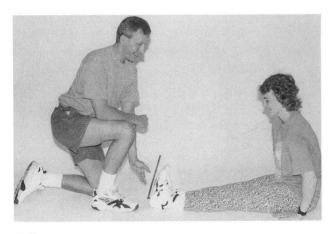

Calf test—pass

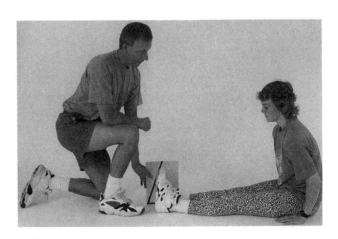

Calf test—fail

WORKSHEET 7A: MUSCULAR ENDURANCE
Curl-Up Tests

The rationale for using curl-ups in place of sit-ups is convincing, and for that reason curl-ups are routinely used in fitness classes. It has taken researchers some time to develop a reliable and valid curl-up test. Presented here are two versions of the test; either may be used. In both cases, the norms listed are based on preliminary data. Test 1 follows the guidelines presented by The Prudential FITNESSGRAM, a program of fitness education and testing designed for grades K–12. Test 2 describes the Robertson Modified Curl-Up Test; its norms were derived from testing college physical education majors. The FITNESSGRAM test requires you to curl up farther. Select one test and follow all the directions.

Equipment:

1. markers—lines taped to the floor or mat or a specially designed curl-up board (See sources listed with norms. If using the tape method, you may want to tape something like a pencil to the floor for the second marker so that the person being tested can feel that she or he has curled up far enough.)

2. metronome or audiocassette for cadence (test 1) or
   stopwatch (test 2)

3. pencil or pen

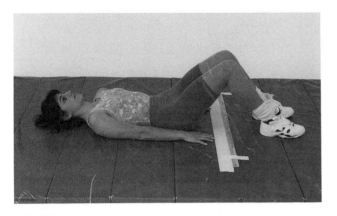

FIGURE A

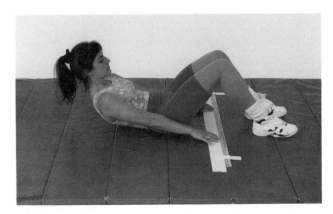

FIGURE B

Specific Directions (differences between tests):

Test 1

Fingertips move 4½ inches

Head touches down between
  curl-ups

Knees bent 140 degrees

Curl to a 3-second cadence
  a maximum of 75 times

Test 2

Fingertips move 3 inches

Shoulder blades touch down between
  curl-ups

Knees bent 90 degrees

Perform as many curls as possible
  in 1 minute

General Directions:

1. Lie on your back with knees bent, arms straight and parallel to your trunk, fingers pointing toward your feet, and palms flat on the floor.

2. Line up fingertips with the initial marker (Figure A).

(continued)

3. Keeping the hips, heels, and fingertips in contact with the floor, curl up until fingertips reach the second marker (Figure B). Fingertips on both hands must simultaneously reach the second marker. You must also breathe throughout the test. Make sure you are adhering to the criteria for the test you selected. Uncurl.

4. Practice the correct technique 5 times.

5. Your partner/instructor will start either the cadence (test 1) or the stopwatch (test 2).

6. Your partner should count correct curl-ups aloud. If you hear a number repeated, you must correct your technique or lose credit for that curl-up.

7. At the end of the test, the starting fingertip position should be rechecked. If you have moved during the test, your score is not valid.

8. Stretch out legs and abdominal muscles.

Test 1. The Prudential FITNESSGRAM standards for healthy fitness zone (age 17+).

	M	F
Score	24–47	18–35

Source: *The Prudential FITNESSGRAM Test Administration Manual.* Dallas, TX: The Cooper Institute for Aerobics Research, 1992. Reprinted with permission.

Test 2. Preliminary norm table based on physical education majors' scores (Northern Illinois University).

PERFORMANCE LEVEL	SCORE	
	M	F
Excellent	103–118	98–115
Good	87–102	80–97
Average	69–86	60–79
Below average	53–68	42–59
Poor	37–52	23–41

Source: Reprinted with permission from the *JOPERD* (*Journal of Physical Education, Recreation, and Dance*), August, 1993, 62–66. *JOPERD* is a publication of the American Alliance for Health, Physical Education, Recreation and Dance, 1900 Association Drive, Reston, VA 22091-1599.

Results:

Number of completed curl-ups: _____

Test 1: _____ I was in the healthy fitness zone.

_____ I was not in the healthy fitness zone.

Test 2: _____ fitness rating.

WORKSHEET 7B: MUSCULAR ENDURANCE
Push-Up Test

Equipment:

1. partner

2. mat or towel (for knees during modified push-ups)

3. pencil or pen

Directions:

1. Warm up and stretch, especially arms and chest.

2. Decide whether you will be performing regular or modified push-ups. (Regular push-ups are performed on hands and toes, modified push-ups are performed on hands and knees.) The norms for modified push-ups are based on a female population, whereas the norms for regular push-ups are based on a male population. (Either gender may perform either test as long as it is understood that so far no norms have been compiled for females doing regular push-ups and males performing modified push-ups.)

3. To begin this test, lie on your stomach, legs together. Position your hands under your shoulders with fingers pointing forward. On the start signal push up from the mat, fully extending your elbows, and then lower down until your chin touches the mat. Your chest and abdomen should not touch the floor. You must maintain a straight body alignment at all times. Your partner will count only correctly completed push-ups.

4. There is no time limit on this test. Perform as many correct push-ups as you can without taking a break. The test will be stopped when you strain forcibly or are unable to maintain correct technique over two repetitions.

5. Record the number of correct push-ups you complete.
   _____ push-ups   Circle one: Regular   Modified

6. Consult the norms below and record your fitness level. (Fill in an "X" if there are no gender-appropriate norms for the test position you selected.)
   _____ fitness rating

7. Stretch your arms and chest muscles to prevent soreness.

Norms by age groups and gender for push-ups.*

FITNESS RATING	AGE (YEARS)											
	15–19		20–29		30–39		40–49		50–59		60–69	
	M	F	M	F	M	F	M	F	M	F	M	F
Excellent	≥39	≥33	≥36	≥30	≥30	≥27	≥22	≥24	≥21	≥21	≥18	≥17
Above Average	29–38	25–32	29–35	21–29	22–29	20–26	17–21	15–23	13–20	11–20	11–17	12–16
Average	23–28	18–24	22–28	15–20	17–21	13–19	13–16	11–14	10–12	7–10	8–10	5–11
Below Average	18–22	12–17	17–21	10–14	12–16	8–12	10–12	5–10	7–9	2–6	5–7	1–4
Poor	≤17	≤11	≤16	≤9	≤11	≤7	≤9	≤4	≤6	≤1	≤4	≤1

*Based on data from the Canada Fitness Survey, 1981.

From: *The Canadian Standardized Test of Fitness—Operations Manual*, 3rd Edition, 1986. Used with permission from the Canadian Society for Exercise Physiology in cooperation with Fitness Canada–Health Canada.

WORKSHEET 8: HEALTHY/IDEAL WEIGHT

Height/Weight Chart

Measure your height in inches:

Measure your weight in pounds:

Cross reference your height, weight, and age on Table 11.3 (see page 107).

My suggested weight is _____ pounds.

Modified Mahoney Formula

(See page 106.)

	Women	Men
Height in inches:	☐	☐
	x 0.35	x 0.40
	☐	☐
	− 108	− 128
Ideal weight:	☐	☐

Ideal Weight Calculated Using Known Percent Fat

(See pages 105–106.)

☐   Present % fat   ☐   Present weight
                                    in pounds

− ☐   Ideal % fat   x   ☐   Decimal form of
                                    % fat difference

☐   Difference in % fat   ☐   Pounds to be lost

÷ 100

☐   Decimal form of   ☐   Present weight in pounds
      % fat difference

                              ☐   Pounds to be lost

                          − ☐   Ideal weight

WORKSHEET 9A: NUTRITION AWARENESS

Record what you eat during one **weekday**.   Date: _____

MEAL:	FOODS ———→	FOOD GROUPS ——→	AMOUNTS/SERVINGS

MEAL:

Breakfast: Time_____

   Time spent eating _____

   Location _____

_____

_____

_____

Lunch: Time_____

   Time spent eating_____

   Location _____

_____

_____

_____

Dinner: Time_____

   Time spent eating_____

   Location _____

_____

_____

_____

Snacks: Time(s)_____

   Time spent eating _____

   Location _____

_____

Alcohol: Time(s)_____

   Time spent drinking _____

Place the total number of servings you ate on this day inside the appropriate food pyramid boxes:

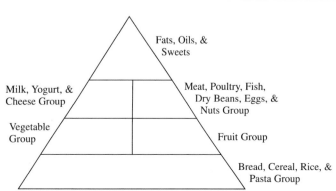

WORKSHEET 9B: NUTRITION AWARENESS

Record what you eat during one **weekend day.**   Date: _____

| **MEAL:** | **FOODS** ⟶ | ⟶**FOOD GROUPS** | ⟶**AMOUNTS/SERVINGS** |

MEAL:
_____

Breakfast: Time _____

   Time spent eating _____

   Location _____

_____

_____

_____

Lunch: Time _____

   Time spent eating _____

   Location _____

_____

_____

_____

Dinner: Time _____

   Time spent eating _____

   Location _____

_____

_____

_____

Snacks: Time(s) _____

   Time spent eating _____

   Location _____

_____

Alcohol: Time(s) _____

   Time spent drinking _____

Place the total number of servings you ate on this day
inside the appropriate food pyramid boxes:

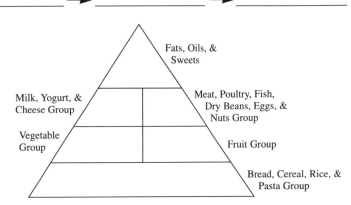

WORKSHEET 9C: NUTRITION AWARENESS

After recording your diet for one day during the week and for one day over the weekend, read and answer the questions below.

1. Did you eat the appropriate number of servings from the food pyramid? If not, which areas need improvement?

Weekday:

Weekend:

2. How many glasses of water (fluids not containing caffeine or alcohol) did you drink? What is recommended for your level of activity? (p. 101)

Weekday: _____   Weekend: _____   Recommended: _____

Are you drinking enough water?   Yes   No

3. What percentage of your total food intake did you eat before dinner? What percentage is recommended? (p. 107)

Weekday: _____   Weekend: _____   Recommended: _____

4. What percentage of your carbohydrates were complex or natural sugar carbohydrates? What percentage is recommended? (p. 100)

Weekday: _____   Weekend: _____   Recommended: _____

5. If you could start the day over, what one thing would you most like to change about your diet?

Weekday:

Weekend:

6. What one thing would you most like to keep the same?

Weekday:

Weekend:

(continued)

7. Did you eat your meals at the same time of day each day? What implications might this have?

8. Other comments or observations:

Index

Abdominals, 71–72
 exercises, 72–75
Adaptations, 92
Addiction to exercise, 16
Adenosine triphosphate (ATP),
 93, 97
Adherence, 25, 97, 98
Aerobic, 16
Aerobic dance; *see also*
 Rhythmic aerobics
 benefits of, 91–98
 defined, 45
 technique, 46–48
Aerobic system, 93
 aerobic glycolysis, 93
 fatty acid oxidation (beta
 oxidation), 93
Aerobic target zone, 15–23;
 see also Target zone
Agonist, 33, 95–96
Amino acids, 100
Anabolic steroids, 97
Anaerobic exercises:
 benefits of, 92–93
 defined, 93
Anaerobic systems, 92–93
 anaerobic glycolysis, 92–93
 phosphagen system, 92
Anorexia, 110
Antagonist, 33, 95–96
Arteries, 19
 capillaries, 94
 carotid, 19–20
 coronary, 94–95, 101
 radial, 19
Arteriosclerosis, 94, 101
Asthma and exercise, 118
Atherosclerosis, 94, 101
Aqua aerobics, 53, 83
 differences from land aerobics,
 54

Back care, 118–119, 137–138

Bands, exercise, 7, 78–83
Baroreceptor, 19
Belts, 6
Bench aerobics, *see* Step aerobics
Blisters, 4, 7, 114
Blood pressure, 93–94
Body composition, 10, 103
 assessing, 105–107
 percent body fat, 105, 106
 weight adjustment and loss,
 107–109
Body toning, 59–62
 with bands, 78
 muscle contractions, 61
 resistance, increasing, 77
 technique, 61
 with water, 83
 with weights, 83–84
Body toning exercises, 62–76,
 78–83
 abdominals, 71–75
 arms and shoulders, 68–71, 75,
 79, 82
 back, 75–76, 80
 with bands and weights, 79–83
 combination, 67–68, 71, 76
 foot and ankle, 4, 82–83
 legs, 61–67, 80–82
 in water, 83
Boredom during exercise, 120
Borg scale, *see* RPE scale
Bra, sports, 6
Bulimia, 110
Burn (lactic acid), 92, 120
Bursitis, 117

Caffeine, 111–112
Calcium, 102
Calluses, 4
Calories, 100
 burning, 108–109
Carbohydrates, 92–93, 100
 aerobic glycolysis, 93

Cardiac output, 93
Cardiorespiratory endurance,
 9–10
 fitness tests, 151–158
Cardiovascular system, 93–94
 benefits of exercise on, 46,
 94–95
 interval training for, 55
Cholesterol, 96, 101
Circuit aerobics, 54–55
Clothing, 1–6
 dangerous, 6
 shoes, *see* Shoes
Cool-down:
 defined, 43
 standing, 43
 stretch, developmental, 44
 stretches, 34–42, 44
Coronary heart disease (CHD),
 101
Cross training, 3–4, 120
Curl-up test, 165–166

Dangerous clothing, 6
Dehydration, 6, 101
Developmental stretch, 44
Diabetes and exercise, 118
Diet; *see also* Nutrition
 fad, 110
 portions, 103
 unbalanced, 110
Dizziness during exercise, 119
Don'ts, *see* Exercises to avoid
Duration, *see* Time

Eating disorders, 110
Electrolytes, replacing, 101
Endorphins, 27
Energy balance, 107
Energy systems, *see* Metabolic
 systems
Equipment:
 bands, exercise, 7, 78–83

mats, exercise, 6
pulse readers, 7
steps (benches), 7, 49
weights, 6–7, 83
Exercise:
    with asthma, 118
    back care during, 118–119
    benefits of, 91–98
    with diabetes, 118
    eating, during and before, 111
    facility, 123–125
    high, 27
    levels, 22
    in pregnancy, 118
    programs, selecting, 28, 45–46,
      123–126
    while sick, 119
Exercise heart rate (EHR):
    chart, 21
    defined, 18
    formula, 18
    worksheet, 149–150
Exercises:
    aerobic dance, *see* Rhythmic
      aerobics
    to avoid, 85–89
    body toning, *see* Body toning
      exercises
    stretching, *see* Stretching
      exercises

Fad diets, 110
Fat, 100–101, 103, 105
    fatty acid oxidation, 93
    intramuscular, 103
    measurement of, 105–107
    metabolism of, 92–93
    percent, *see* Body composition
    saturated, 101
    subcutaneous, 10, 103
    unsaturated, 101
FIT, 12; *see also* Target zone
Fitness:
    goals, *see* Goals
    target zone, *see* Target zone
    tests, *see* Tests
Fitness components, 9–11; *see
    also individual items as
    main entries*
    body composition, 10
    cardiorespiratory endurance, 10
    flexibility, 10

muscular endurance, 10–11
    muscular strength, 11
    skill-related, 10
Flexibility; *see also* Stretching;
    benefits, 10, 32
    defined, 10
    fitness tests, 159–163
    target zone, 32–33
Food guide pyramid, 102–103,
    171–173
Food serving, 103
Foot injuries:
    blisters, 4, 7, 114
    bunions, 114
    calluses, 4
    metatarsalgia, 114
    Morton's neuroma, 115
    plantar fascitis, 114
Frequency (component of FIT):
    aerobic training target zone,
      15–16
    defined, 11–12
    flexibility target zone, 32
    muscular strength and endur-
      ance target zone, 60

Glucose, 100, 101
Glycogen, 100
Goals, 25–30
    evaluating, 29–30
    long-range, 27
    measuring, 28–29
    realistic, 26–27
    short-range, 27
    specific, 26
Golgi tendon organ, 96

Health-related fitness, 9–11
Heart rate (HR), 16–21
    chart, 21
    defined, 17
    formulas, 17–19
    to monitor intensity of
      exercise, 17, 20, 22
    pulse, 19–20
    worksheets, 145–150
Heart rate reserve
    (HR_{max}reserve), 16–18
    benefits from aerobics, 120
    defined, 18
    formula, 18
    target zone, 22–23

worksheet, 149–150
Heat:
    cramp, *see* Muscle cramp
    exhaustion, 117
    stroke, 117–118
Height/weight chart, 107
High-density lipoproteins (HDL),
    95, 101
High-impact aerobics (HIA),
    45–48
Homeostasis, 92, 93
Hydrostatic weighing, 105
Hyperextension, 85–89
Hypertrophy, 96, 97

Ideal weight, *see* Weight
Impact stress, *see* Stress
Impedance machine (body
    analyzer), 105
Individuality, principle of, 12
Injuries, 113
    bursitis, 117
    foot, 114–115
    heat exhaustion, 117
    heat stroke, 117–118
    knee, 115–116
    low-impact aerobics to prevent,
      48–49
    muscle cramp, 117, 119
    prevention, 47, 114
    shin, 115
    sprain, 116
    strain, 116
    stress, *see* Stress
    tendinitis, 116–117
Intensity (component of FIT):
    aerobic training target zone,
      16–22
    defined, 11–12
    flexibility target zone, 32–33
    muscular strength and endur-
      ance target zone, 60
Interval training, 55
Iron, 102
Isometric contractions, 11, 61
Isotonic contractions, 11, 61

Karvonen formula, 17–19,
    147–148; *see also* Training
    heart rate range
Knee injuries:
    chondromalacia patella, 115

meniscal, 116

Lactic acid system, 93
Lean body mass (LBM), 103; *see also* Body composition
Leotards, 5–6
Levels of exercise, 22
Ligaments, 4
Low-density lipoproteins (LDL), 101
Low-impact aerobics (LIA), 15, 48–49

Mats, exercise, 6
Maximum heart rate (HRmax):
    defined, 17
    formulas, 17–19
    worksheet, 145–146
Maximum oxygen uptake, 16
Medical history, 141–142
Metabolic systems, 92–93
Minerals, 102
Motivation, 27–28
    sources of, 28
Muscle:
    agonist and antagonist, 33, 95–96
    spindle, 96
Muscle contractions:
    concentric, 96
    dynamic, 11
    eccentric, 96
    isometric, 11
    isotonic, 11
Muscle cramp, 117, 119
Muscular strength and endurance:
    benefits, 11
    defined, 10–11, 59
    exercises, *see* Body toning exercises
    fitness tests, 165–167
    target zone, 60–61
    technique, 61
Muscular system:
    benefits of exercise on, described, 95–96
    pictured, 136

Nervous system:
    benefits of exercise on, 97
    described, 97
Norms, 12, 28–29

Nutrition, 99–103
    carbohydrates, 100
    fat, 100–101; *see also* Fat
    food label, interpreting, 104
    food pyramid, 102–103
    minerals, 102
    protein, 100
    vitamins, 102
    water, 101–102, 111
    worksheets, 169–176

Obesity, 105
Orthotics, 2, 4
Osteoporosis, 95
Overfat, 103
Overload, principle of, 11
Overtraining, 16, 119
Overuse, principle of, 13
Overweight, 103
Oxygen consumption, 16

Percent fat, *see* Body composition
Phosphagen system, 92
PNF stretching, 33, 96
Posture, 95
Pre-exercise heart rate (PreHR):
    chart, 21
    defined, 20
    worksheet, 149–150
Pregnancy, 118, 124
Principles of exercise:
    FIT, *see* Target zone
    individuality, 12
    overload, 11
    overuse, 13
    progression, 12
    reversibility, 12
    specificity, 12
    use/disuse, 12
Progression, principle of, 12
Proprioceptive neuromuscular facilitation (PNF stretching), 33, 96
Protein, 100
Psychological benefits of exercise, 97–98
Pulse, *see also* Heart rate
    defined, 17
    monitoring, frequency of, 11
    monitoring, how to, 17–19
    readers, 7
    sites, 19

Push-up test, 167

Range of motion, 10, 32
Rating of perceived exertion, *see* RPE scale
Recovery heart rate (RecHR):
    defined, 20
    chart, 21
    worksheet, 149–150
Respiratory system:
    benefits of exercise on, 95
    described, 95
Reproductive system:
    benefits of exercise on, 97
    described, 97
Resting heart rate (RHR), 16–20
    benefits of aerobics, 94
    defined, 17
    formula, 18
    worksheets, 145–150
Reversibility, principle of, 12
Rhythmic aerobics, 45–58; *see also individual items as main entries*
    aqua (water), 53–54
    circuit, 54–55
    defined, 45–46
    high-impact (HIA), 47–48
    low-impact (LIA), 48–49
    slide, 55–58
    step (bench), 49–53
    techniques for, 46–47
    videotapes, 58
RICE, 121
Risk of injury, reducing, *see* Injuries
RPE scale, 20, 22

Shin injuries:
    shinsplints, 113, 115
    stress fractures, 115
Shoes, 1–4
    aerobic vs. running, 4
    guidelines for selecting, 4
    parts of, 2–3
    support, arch, 3
    support, lateral, 3
Shorts, 6
Skeletal system:
    benefits of exercise on, 95
    described, 95
Skin-fold technique, 105–106

Slide aerobics, 55
  basic movements, 56–57
  techniques, 58
Socks, 4–5
  warmup, 6
Specificity, principle of, 12
Spot reducing, 111
Sprain, 116
Step (bench) aerobics, 7, 49, 53
  basic movements, 50–52
  techniques, 53
Step tests, 151–154
Strain, 116
Strength, *see* Muscular strength
Stress:
  fracture, 115
  impact, 1–4, 46–49
  injuries, 49
  minimizing, 15
Stretch:
  cool-down, *see* Cool-down
  developmental, 44
  reflex, 96
  warm-up, *see* Warm-up
Stretching:
  antagonist, 33
  assisted (passive), 33
  ballistic, 32, 96
  bounce, 32
  proprioceptive neuromuscular
    facilitation (PNF), 33, 96
  static, 32, 96
Stretching exercises:
  abdominal, 36, 42
  back, 36, 42
  legs, 37–43
  neck, 34

shoulder, 35
Stroke volume, 93
Sweat, 119

Target zone:
  aerobic, 15–16, 22
  cardiorespiratory endurance,
    11, 22
  defined, 11–12
  FIT, 11–12, 15–17, 22–23
  fitness, 11
  flexibility, 32–33
  heart rate, *see* Training heart
    rate range
  muscular strength and endur-
    ance, 60–61
  pulse, 19–20
Tendinitis, 116, 117
Tests, 28–29
  assessing body composition,
    105–107
  cardiorespiratory fitness,
    151–158
  flexibility, 159–163
  hydrostatic weighing, 105
  muscular endurance, 165–167
  skin-fold, 105
  summary worksheet, 143–144
  table, 29
Threshold of training:
  aerobic, 16–17
  defined, 11
Tights, 5
Time (component of FIT):
  aerobic target zone, 16
  defined, 11–12
  flexibility target zone, 32

muscular strength and endurance target zone, 60
Training heart rate range (THR),
  16–23, 120–121
  defined, 17
  formulas, 17–19
  worksheets, 145–150

Undergarments for women, 6
Underwater weighing, 105
Use/disuse, principle of, 12

Venous pump, 43
Vitamins, 102
VO_2max, 16

Walk–run tests, 155–157
Warm-up:
  core, 31–32
  defined, 31
  stretches, 33–43
  stretch techniques, 31–33
  technique tips, 32
Water, 101–102, 111
Water aerobics, *see* Aqua aerobics
Weight:
  adjustment, 107–109
  calculating healthy, 106
  control, 103, 105–112
  diets, 110
  gain, 109
  healthy vs. ideal, 106–107, 109
  loss, 107–111
  maintenance, 109
Weights, 6–7, 83